Improving Outcomes in Chronic Heart Failure

Sp

re

The editors dedicate this book to Dr Caroline Morrison whose dedication and support enabled the Glasgow service to be set up.

Improving Outcomes in Chronic Heart Failure

Specialist nurse intervention from research to practice

Edited by

Simon Stewart

National Heart Foundation of Australia/Roche Chair of Cardiovascular Nursing, University of South Australia, Australia

Lynda Blue

Nurse Coordinator, Heart Failure Liaison Service, Greater Glasgow Primary Care NHS Trust, Glasgow, Scotland

First published in 2004
by BMJ Books, BMA House, Tavistock Square,
London WC1H 9JR

First edition published in 2001 as Improving Outcomes in Chronic Heart
Failure: a practical guide to specialist nurse interventions

www.bmjbooks.com

British Library Cataloguing in Publication Data

A catalogue record for this book is available from the British Library

ISBN 0 7279 1723 4

Typeset by SIVA Math Setters, Chennai, India
Printed and bound by in Spain by GraphyCems, Navarra

Contents

Contributors

Lynda Blue
Nurse Coordinator, Heart Failure Liaison Service, Greater Glasgow Primary Care NHS Trust, Glasgow, Scotland

John Carson
Heart Failure Liaison Nurse, Victoria Infirmary, Glasgow, Scotland

Alison Freeman
Area Clinical Effectiveness Facilitator, Department of Public Health, Greater Glasgow NHS Board, Glasgow, Scotland

Eric Gray
Heart Failure Liaison Nurse, Western Infirmary, Glasgow, Scotland

Laura Mackintosh
Heart Failure Liaison Nurse, Stobhill Hospital, Glasgow, Scotland

Margaret B McEntegart
British Heart Foundation Cardiology Research Fellow, Department of Cardiology, University of Glasgow/Western Infirmary, Glasgow, Scotland

Linda McGinnis
Heart Failure Liaison Nurse, Southern General Hospital, Glasgow, Scotland

Iona McKay
Heart Failure Liaison Nurse, Western Infirmary, Glasgow, Scotland

John McMurray
Professor of Medical Cardiology and Honorary Consultant Cardiologist, Department of Cardiology, Western Infirmary, Glasgow, Scotland

Yvonne Millerick
Heart Failure Liaison Nurse, Glasgow Royal Infirmary, Glasgow, Scotland

Kirstie Mowat
Heart Failure Liaison Nurse, Southern General Hospital, Glasgow, Scotland

Katriona Mullen
Heart Failure Liaison Nurse, Victoria Infirmary, Glasgow, Scotland

Kirstin Russell
Heart Failure Liaison Nurse, Glasgow Royal Infirmary, Glasgow, Scotland

Simon Stewart
National Heart Foundation of Australia/Roche Chair of Cardiovascular Nursing, University of South Australia, Australia

Foreword

Since the publication of the first edition of this text, we have made a number of discoveries that have improved the care of patients with heart failure. The debate about the clinical and economic benefits of systematic heart failure programs is over. The data are irrefutable related to the short- and long-term benefits of such programs. Moreover, clinical trials have given us new information about the utility of new classes of drugs and surgical approaches in the treatment of this life-threatening chronic illness that has made care more effective.

Despite the advances in science, the challenges in heart failure care remain just as daunting as they were when the first edition of this text was published. Heart failure remains a major health problem for millions of individuals around the world. It is the number one cause of hospitalisation in elderly patients in many industrialised countries. It remains a leading cause of morbidity and mortality, and is increasingly prevalent in developing countries, quickly overcoming infectious disease and malnutrition as a cause of mortality. Many clinicians have come to realise that the best, most cutting edge treatments are ineffective without the active involvement of the patient and family.

This second edition retains many of its unique characteristics. Firstly, it continues to be the only textbook on heart failure that presents an international, multidisciplinary perspective. The editors have gathered experts from many countries and different disciplines to consider the issues surrounding the care of patients with heart failure. Given the different cultures and healthcare systems represented, the innovative and creative approaches to heart failure treatment offered in these pages hold great promise.

Secondly, the book goes well beyond the usual discussion of epidemiology, diagnosis and treatment. It provides critical insight into the elements required of a heart failure clinical service, incorporating recent experiences of nurse specialists. The majority of patients with heart failure are cared for in traditional medical practices, without the benefit of a systematic nursing approach. Healthcare providers interested in instituting such a service will find these pages highly useful. The authors provide excellent descriptions of the core elements of such a programme, as well as successful examples.

Thirdly, the text retains its commitment to interdisciplinary care. The histories of the healthcare professions combined with the constraints of many healthcare systems can, at times, present difficult barriers to organising an interdisciplinary heart failure programme.

However, the full participation of the entire team – nurse, physician, pharmacist, dietician, and others – is critical to the ultimate success of treatment. The authors describe a nurse-led, interdisciplinary approach that is now recognised as the key to successful heart failure management. They have also included the details required to reduce traditional barriers and begin a successful heart failure service.

This highly readable text incorporates the latest science and is an important contribution to the literature. Ultimately our patients will be the beneficiaries.

Preface

So much has happened since we compiled the first edition of this book – *Improving outcomes in chronic heart failure: a practial guide to specialist nurse intervention*. Heart failure as a truly malignant, debilitating, and costly syndrome has finally attracted the kind of attention and resources it deserves in many developed countries. With this attention has come an increasing awareness that without a legitimate and widely available cure, our best efforts merely prolong an inevitable but often unpredictable decline in the functional status and quality of life of patients with this syndrome. It is within this essentially grim context that the evidence for applying predominantly nurse-led programmes of care designed to optimise the management of patients who have been hospitalised with chronic heart failure has been strengthened considerably and the number of funded programmes has risen exponentially. Unlike when the first edition was published, there are now few academics or clinicians who would argue against the widespread application of specific programmes of heart failure care in order to cost-effectively reduce recurrent readmissions, improve quality of life, and perhaps prolong survival in typically older patients in whom treatment options are limited and/or difficult to apply.

This "good news" has to be tempered, however, with the realisation that some things have not changed. For example, without a cure, the prevalence of heart failure continues to rise and predictions of a sustained epidemic in the 21st century are still well founded with little relief in sight. Given the ongoing individual and societal burden imposed by heart failure, therefore, it is disappointing to note that despite the wealth of evidence and its incorporation into expert heart failure treatment guidelines, the types of programme described in our first edition are still not widely applied. Part of the problem is undoubtedly cost considerations within financially stressed healthcare systems. Another problem is a lack of appreciation of the depth of evidence from a wide range of countries to support the application of nurse-led heart failure programmes of care. Finally and most importantly, there is the widespread problem of "good intent" and funding to apply heart failure programmes without specific information and expertise to actually implement the evidence in an expert manner.

It is within this context and in acknowledgement of the limitations of the first edition in providing a preliminary guide to establishing nurse-led programmes of care that we present this second edition, appropriately entitled *Improving outcomes in chronic heart failure:*

specialist nurse intervention from research to practice. Consistent with our promise to the many healthcare professionals who have sought our advice these past few years, this second edition provides a firm financial argument for funding such programmes of care and, most importantly, concentrates on the practical implications of providing a comprehensive service with realistic case scenarios and advice on how to apply the evidence from recent clinical trials (for example CHARM, COPERNICUS, MERIT, CIBIS II and RALES) into clinical practice.

Naturally, we are biased in our preference for incorporating home visits into any management programme and we are delighted to include the contributions of the expert nurses who are part of the now world-renowned Glasgow Heart Failure Liaison Service in Scotland. However, we firmly believe that any clinician or administrator with an interest in applying this type of programme of care will find a wealth of practical and informative guidance in this book.

In conclusion, we wish you well in your endeavours to improve the lives of those unfortunate enough to develop or be affected by chronic heart failure and hope this book provides the inspiration and advice to apply an effective programme of care and make a tangible difference to many people's lives.

Simon Stewart
Lynda Blue

Section 1:
Background

1: Increased health care utilisation and costs: heart failure in the 21st century

SIMON STEWART

Introduction

In a world of mixed messages and confusing statistics it is often difficult to grasp the enormity of a particular problem until it reaches overwhelming proportions. For example our relative success in steadily reducing cardiovascular-related mortality rates,[1] predominantly via improved treatment and prevention of an acute myocardial infarction and sudden cardiac death,[2] has blinded many to the paradoxical and dramatic increase in older individuals with underlying heart disease (in most cases there is no cure) at risk of developing a severe form of chronic heart disease.

Chronic heart failure, a disabling and deadly syndrome that typically represents the end product of a lifetime of "insults" to the structural integrity and efficiency of the heart, is one such clinical problem that is only now receiving the type of recognition and response that it deserves. Certainly, clinicians who are aware of the enormous flow-on effect of trying to manage even a few old and fragile patients with chronic heart failure are under no illusion as to its current impact on healthcare systems around the globe – similar to the ripples that emanate from a single stone dropped into a still pond, heart failure reaches out to disrupt the lives of those living directly and indirectly with this truly malignant syndrome and also severely impairs the capacity of the local healthcare system to cope with other health priorities.

We now know that in the geographic regions of Europe (6·5 million), Japan (2·4 million), the USA (5 million) and Australia (0·4 million) a combined total of almost 15 million people are directly affected by chronic heart failure.[3] It is within this context that this introductory chapter provides an overview of an evolving epidemic of international proportions. Specifically, it outlines the key epidemiological features of heart failure with particular emphasis on the likely impact it will have on healthcare systems in the foreseeable future. It goes on to demonstrate how best it can be cost-effectively tackled to both relieve individual suffering and reduce the enormous burden it imposes on progressively ageing populations as a whole.

Defining the burden of heart failure

When describing the burden imposed by chronic heart failure it is important to acknowledge two significant limitations. First, heart failure represents a complex pathological process that is the terminal manifestation of a number of diverse but often interrelated cardiac disease states. These often include coronary heart disease and chronic systolic hypertension. As such, it is associated with a broad spectrum of clinical presentations and defies simple definition. The most practical of definitions comes from the European Society of Cardiology, that defines chronic heart failure as:

> Symptoms of heart failure at rest or on effort, combined with objective evidence of cardiac dysfunction at rest, together with a response to treatment directed towards heart failure.[4]

Second, our understanding of heart failure has largely relied on epidemiological studies (most of those listed in Table 1.1) that have lacked an objective measure of cardiac dysfunction. Fortunately, the relative dearth of large-scale, systematic investigations of the epidemiology of chronic heart failure from both a physiological and a clinical perspective within the same population has been addressed in recent times (see Table 1.2). These studies, whilst difficult to interpret given the range of criteria used to confirm the presence of "objective evidence of cardiac dysfunction", have highlighted the large number of asymptomatic individuals within the population who might be legitimately labelled with a diagnosis of "latent heart failure" (for example those with asymptomatic left ventricular systolic dysfunction). They also indicate the presence of a large number of individuals who have symptoms of heart failure derived from cardiac dysfunction without evidence of impaired left ventricular systolic dysfunctions (so called "diastolic" heart failure).

In most cases symptomatic heart failure is usually characterised by the following:

- left ventricular dysfunction (systolic or diastolic)
- abnormal neurohormonal regulation
- unmet metabolic demand
- breathlessness and intolerance to exercise
- fluid retention
- premature death.

Data relating to the aetiology, epidemiology, and prognostic implications of chronic heart failure are principally available from five types of studies:

- cross-sectional and longitudinal follow-up surveys of well-defined populations: these have almost exclusively focused on individuals with clinical signs and symptoms indicative of chronic congestive heart failure
- cross-sectional surveys of individuals who have been medically treated for signs and symptoms of heart failure within a well-defined region
- echocardiograph surveys of individuals within a well-defined population to determine the prevalence of left ventricular systolic dysfunction
- national studies of annual trends in hospitalisation related to heart failure identified on the basis of diagnostic coding at discharge
- comprehensive clinical trial and trial registry datasets: these include a large proportion of individuals who were identified on the basis of having both impaired left ventricular systolic dysfunction and signs and symptoms of heart failure.

The overall burden imposed by heart failure on any given health-care system can be estimated by combining such information with specific cost–utilisation data. Furthermore, by analysing trends in the common precursors of heart failure in addition to the epidemiological parameters and related health care utilisation rates it is possible to predict the likely burden imposed by heart failure in the longer term.

Within the context of the specific limitations of the type of data available and the inherent bias towards describing chronic congestive heart failure secondary to left ventricular systolic dysfunction, the following sections describe the modern-day burden of chronic heart failure and its likely impact in the longer term.

The burden imposed by heart failure

Prevalence of heart failure within the general population

Table 1.1 is a summary of the reported prevalence of heart failure according to whether this was estimated from a survey of individuals requiring medical treatment from a general practitioner, or from population screening. Despite the wide variation in the overall prevalence of heart failure reported (largely reflecting different research methodologies and study cohorts), these data demonstrate that the prevalence of heart failure increases markedly with age and that it has become more common in the last few decades of the 20th century.

Table 1.1 Reported prevalence of heart failure

Study	Location	Prevalence rate, whole population (/1000)	Prevalence rate in older age groups (/1000)
Surveys of treated patients			
Logan et al. (1958)[5]	National data (RCGP), UK	3	–
Gibson et al. (1966)[6]	Rural cohort, USA	9–10	65 (> 65 yr)
RCGP (1988)[7]	National data, UK	11	–
Parameshwar et al. (1992)[8]	London, UK	4	28 (> 65 yr)
Rodeheffer (1993)[9]	Rochester, USA	3 (< 75 yr)	–
Mair et al. (1996)[10]	Liverpool, UK	15	80 (> 65yr)
RCGP (1995)[11]	National data, UK	9	74 (65–74 yr)
Clarke et al. (1995)[12]	Nottinghamshire, UK	8–16	40–60 (> 70 yr)
Population screening			
Droller and Pemberton (1953)[13]	Sheffield, UK	–	30–50 (> 62 yr)
Garrison et al. (1966)[14]	Georgia, USA	21 (45–74 yr)	35 (65–74 yr)
McKee et al. (1971)[15]	Framingham, USA	3 (< 63 yrs)	23 (60–79 yr)
Landahl et al. (1984)[16]	Sweden (males only)	3 (< 75 yr)	80–170 (> 67 yr)
Eriksson et al. (1989)[17]	Gothenburg, Sweden	–	130 (> 67 yr)
Schocken et al.[18]	NHANES data, USA	20	80 (> 65 yr)
RCGP (1995)[11]	National data, UK	9 (25–74 yr)	74 (65–74 yr)

Studies of patients visiting a general practitioner

In the UK there have been a number of large studies examining the prevalence of patients being treated for heart failure by a general practitioner. For example in 1992, Parameshwar and colleagues[8] examined the clinical records of diuretic-treated patients in three general practices in north-west London. From a total of 30 204 patients, a clinical diagnosis of heart failure was made in 117 cases (46 men and 71 women), giving an overall prevalence rate of 3·9 cases per 1000. Prevalence increased markedly with age – in those aged under 65 years the prevalence rate was 0·6 cases per 1000 compared with 28 cases per 1000 in those aged over 65 years. However, objective investigation of left ventricular function had been undertaken in less than one third of these patients. In 1995, Clarke and colleagues[12] reported an even larger survey of chronic heart failure based on similar methods and including analysis of loop diuretic prescriptions for all residents of Nottinghamshire. They estimated that between 13 017 and 26 214 patients had been prescribed furosemide. Case-note review of a random sample of patients receiving such treatment found that 56% were being treated for heart failure. On this basis an overall prevalence rate was calculated of 8–16 per 1000. Once again, prevalence increased with advancing age, with the rate increasing to 40–60 cases per 1000 among those aged over 70 years.

Population studies based on clinical criteria

The National Health and Nutrition Examination Survey (NHANES-I)[18] reported the prevalence of heart failure within the US population. Based on self-reporting, and using a clinical scoring system, this study screened 14 407 men and women aged 25–47 years between 1971 and 1975, with detailed evaluation of only 6913 subjects and reported a prevalence rate of 20 cases per 1000. The Helsinki Ageing Study described clinical and echocardiographic findings in 501 subjects (367 female) aged 75–86 years (see Table 1.2).[26] Prevalence of heart failure, based on clinical criteria, was 8·2% overall (41 of 501) and 6·8%, 10%, and 8·1% in those aged 75, 80 and 85 years respectively. As might be expected in an elderly population with a clinical diagnosis of heart failure, there was a high prevalence of moderate or severe mitral or aortic valvular disease (51%), ischaemic heart disease (54%), and hypertension (54%). However, of the 41 subjects with "heart failure", only 11 had significant left ventricular systolic dysfunction (diagnosed by fractional shortening or left ventricular dilation) and in 20 subjects no echocardiographic abnormality was identified. Despite this, the four-year relative risks of all-cause and cardiovascular mortality associated with chronic heart failure in this population were 2·1 and 4·2, respectively.

Prevalence of impaired or preserved left ventricular systolic function

There are inherent limitations in defining heart failure on the basis of clinical signs and symptoms in the absence of determining the presence or absence of underlying structural or functional heart disease. Furthermore it is recognised that heart failure is not necessarily confined to those with impaired systolic dysfunction but can arise when systolic function appears to be *preserved* (so-called diastolic heart failure). As a result an increasing number of epidemiological studies that have directly measured cardiac function

7

Table 1.2 Proportion of people with symptomatic or asymptomatic left ventricular systolic dysfunction, or normal/preserved left ventricular systolic function in epidemiological studies of heart failure[19-33]

Location	Number of people	Age range (years)	Mean age (years)	Definition of LVSD	Prevalence of LVSD (%)	Proportion symptom-free (%)
Glasgow (Scotland)[19]	1640	25–74	50	LVEF ≤ 30%	2·9	48
				LVEF ≤ 35%	7·7	77
Birmingham (England)[20]	3960	> 45	61	LVEF < 40%	1·8	47
Poole (England)[21]	817	70–84	76	LVEF < 50%	5·3	61
				Mild*	5·0	
				Moderate*	1·6	
				Severe*	0·7	17†
				Any*	7·5	62†
Rotterdam (the Netherlands)[22]	1698	55–95	65	FS ≤ 25%	3·7	60
Västerås (Sweden)[23]	433	75	75	LVEF < 43%	8·9	
				LVWMI < 1·7%	6·8	46
Augsburg (Germany)[24]	1866	25–75	50	LVEF < 48%	2·7	42
Various-CHS (USA)[25]	5201	65–100	73	Abnormal*	3·7	
Helsinki (Finland)[26]	501	75–86		FS < 25%	11·3	79
Various SHS (USA)[27]	3184	45–74	60	Mild (LVEF 40–54%)	11·1	95†
				Severe (LVEF < 40%)	2·9	72†
Copenhagen (Denmark)[28]	2158	≥50		LVWMI ≤ 1·5 or FS < 0·26	2·9	34
Asturias (Spain)[29]	351	≥40	60	LVEF < 50%	3·1	36

(Continued)

Table 1.2 Continued

Location	Number of people	Age range (years)	Mean age (years)	Prevalence of CHF (%)	Proportion with normal/preserved LV systolic function (%)
Helsinki (Finland)[30]	501	75–86		8·2	51**
Various CHS (USA)[31]	4842	66–103	78	8·8	55
Poole (England)[21]	817	70–84	76	7·5	68[†]
Västerås (Sweden)[23]	433	75	75	6·7	46
Rotterdam (the Netherlands)[22]	1698	55–95	65	2·1	71
Various-SHS (USA)[25]	3184	47–81	60	3·0	53
Asturias (Spain)[29]	391	≥40	60	4·9	59
Framingham (USA)[31]	73		73	NA[§]	51
Olmsted County (USA)[32]	137		77	NA[ǁ]	43
Portugal[33]	5434	> 25	68	4·4	39

*Qualitative/semiquantitative assessment of left ventricular systollic function. [†]No self-reported history of heart failure. [‡]No heart failure. [§] Patients with heart failure, nested case–control study. [ǁ]Incidence study. **Excluding patients with valve disease. CHS = Cardiovascular Health Study; FS = fractional shortening of the left ventricle; LV = left ventricular; LVEF = left ventricular ejection fraction; LVWMI = left ventricular wall motion index; NA = not applicable; SHS = Strong Heart Study (American Indians).

have been undertaken. Studies that have reported some form of objective measure are summarised in Table 1.2. In most cases these studies have estimated left ventricular ejection fraction via echocardiography.

Three notable estimates of the population prevalence of left ventricular systolic dysfunction as determined by echocardiography have emanated from Scotland,[19] England[21] and the Netherlands.[22] The Scottish study targeted a representative cohort of 2000 persons aged 25–74 years. Of those selected, 1640 (82%) had a detailed assessment of their cardiovascular status and underwent echocardiography. Left ventricular systolic dysfunction was defined as a left ventricular ejection fraction of 30% or less. The overall prevalence of left ventricular systolic dysfunction using this criterion was 2·9%. Concurrent symptoms of heart failure were found in 1·5% of the cohort, whilst the remaining 1·4% were found to be asymptomatic. Prevalence was greater in men and increased with age (in men aged 65–74 years it was 6·4% and in age-matched women it was 4·9%).[19] The Rotterdam study in the Netherlands, though examining individuals aged 55–74 years, reported similar findings. Overall the prevalence of left ventricular systolic dysfunction, defined in this case as fractional shortening of 25% or less, was 5·5% in men and 2·2% in women.[22] More recently, Morgan and colleagues[21] studied 817 individuals aged 70–84 years selected from two general practices in Southampton, England. Left ventricular function was assessed qualitatively as normal, or as mild, moderate, or severe dysfunction. The overall prevalence of all grades of dysfunction was 7·5% (95% CI 5·8 to 9·5%). Prevalence of left ventricular dysfunction doubled between the age ranges of 70–74 years and over 80 years.

Hospitalisation rates

Some of the most reliable epidemiological data on heart failure come from reports of hospital admissions on a country-by-country basis; although these need to be interpreted with some caution owing to their retrospective nature, variations in coding practices, and changing admission thresholds over time. It is important to note that reports from diverse countries such as Scotland,[34] Spain,[35] the USA,[36,37] Sweden,[38] New Zealand,[39] and the Netherlands[40] relating to the period 1978–1994 showed that heart failure related admission rates were increasing. For example studies undertaken in the UK suggest that 0·2% of the population in the early 1990s were hospitalised for heart failure per annum, and that such admissions accounted for more than 5% of adult general medicine and geriatric hospital admissions – outnumbering those associated with acute myocardial infarction.[34] In the USA heart failure is the most common cause of hospitalisation in people over the age of 65 years.[37]

Preliminary reports from Scotland[41] and the Netherlands,[42] now supported by similar data from Singapore[43] and Sweden,[44] suggest that the population rate of admissions associated with a primary diagnosis of heart failure has begun to plateau. However, there is little doubt that age-adjusted admission rates in older individuals continue to rise and the absolute number of admissions, as a reflection of older societies overall, will also rise (see below).

Overall, the duration of hospital stay associated with chronic heart failure is frequently prolonged and in many cases is rapidly followed by readmission. For example in the UK the mean length of stay for a heart failure related hospitalisation in 1990 was 11·4 days on acute medical wards and 28·5 days on acute geriatric wards.[34] Within the UK about one third of patients are readmitted within 12 months of discharge, whilst the same proportion are reported to be readmitted within 6 months in the USA.[36,37] Such readmission rates are usually higher than for other major causes of hospitalisation, including stroke, hip fracture, and respiratory disease.[45] A recent comparison of readmission rates associated with a number of conditions in three states in the USA and three European countries has highlighted the difficulty in comparing different regions due to confounding variables.[46] However, as expected, chronic heart failure, along with chronic pulmonary disease, was associated with the highest readmission rates in both the US and Europe. Significantly, this study found a clear inverse correlation between index length of stay and readmission rates. In essence, it was found that the shorter the initial length of stay the higher the readmission rate.[46] Although a specific study related to heart failure of institutional variations in readmission and mortality rates did not find such an association when adjusting for a limited number of potential confounders,[47] both studies highlight the importance of evaluating such data on a national and more specifically local level.

Cost of heart failure

In the 1990s it was estimated that the overall cost of managing heart failure consumed a significant amount (1–2%) of healthcare expenditure in developed countries.[48] Not surprisingly, hospitalisations represent the costliest (more than two thirds) component of such expenditure. Given the likelihood of an increasing number (if not population rates) of heart failure related hospitalisations in these countries, it is likely that these reported estimates fall short of the current burden imposed by heart failure.

Data from the UK best illustrate the increasing cost of heart failure in developed countries. In 1990 heart failure was estimated to cost 1·3% of healthcare expenditure.[45] Based on a more contemporary

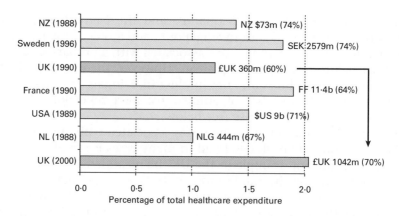

Figure 1.1 The cost of chronic heart failure compared with total healthcare expenditure in six industrialised countries (two estimates for the UK are highlighted)

Percentages shown in parentheses represent the proportion of expenditure relating to hospital-based costs (FF, French francs; NLG, Netherlands guilders; SEK, Swedish kronor; b, billion; m, million).

estimate, for the year 2000, it is now estimated to consume approximately 2·1% of expenditure (based on 1990 equivalent expenditure levels) and, when the cost of hospitalisation associated with a secondary diagnosis of heart failure is also considered, this figure rises markedly to 4%.[49] Figure 1.1 shows the estimated cost of heart failure in a range of developed countries and compares the two estimates derived from the UK a decade apart.

Prognostic implications of chronic heart failure

Chronic heart failure, irrespective of whether it has been detected in patients being actively treated (for example during hospitalisation) or in otherwise asymptomatic individuals, is a lethal condition. Mortality rates may be comparable to that of cancer. For example in the original and subsequent Framingham cohorts, the probability of someone dying within five years of being diagnosed with heart failure was 62% and 75% in men and 38% and 42% in women respectively. In comparison, five-year survival for all cancers among men and women in the USA during the same period was approximately 50%.[50]

These US-derived data clearly suggested that the prognosis in heart failure was often worse than that related to many forms of cancer. Although such a comparison may appear to be clinically redundant there was a clear recognition that raising the awareness of the poor

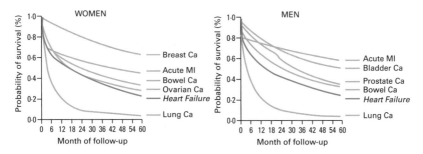

Figure 1.2 Comparison of five-year survival curves: chronic heart failure versus acute myocardial infarction and the most common forms of cancer

prognosis associated with heart failure would facilitate attempts to raise awareness of the enormous impact heart failure imposes on whole populations.

Population based data

It was within this context that, in a recently reported study examining the whole Scottish population, five-year survival rates for all patients admitted for the first time with heart failure in 1991 were directly compared to those patients admitted for the first time with the most common types of cancer (specific to men and women) in addition to acute myocardial infarction.[51] Figure 1.2 shows the crude five-year survival rates for each diagnosis, suggesting that heart failure is at least as "malignant" as cancer and, as expected, has a worse prognosis than a first acute myocardial infarction. Multivariate analysis showed that, with the major exception of lung cancer, heart failure was associated with the poorest longer-term adjusted survival in men. In women both cancer of the breast and large bowel were associated with better short-term survival rates in comparison to heart failure. Subsequent long-term survival was more favourable in the former and equivalent in the latter. Alternatively, cancer of the ovary and lung were associated with poorer adjusted survival rates overall in comparison to heart failure.

Consistent with more recent data from the Framingham Study,[52] it was found that heart failure was associated with a significant number of "premature" life years lost (on average nine years per person), being associated with more deaths than the combination of large bowel, prostate, and bladder cancer. In women, despite the fact that proportionately more deaths occurred in those who had already exceeded average life expectancy, heart failure was second only to myocardial infarction in terms of the total number of premature deaths. Both lung and breast cancer, however, by virtue of a greater number of expected life years lost per person, had a greater impact on the population as a whole during this period.[51]

Overall, these Scottish data[51] support those from the US-based Framingham cohort,[52] a similar report from Ontario, Canada that mirrored the approach used in the Scottish study,[53] and the contemporary UK-based population cohort from London[54] suggesting that heart failure survival rates, in both men and women, are comparable to or even worse than those associated with cancer. These data also provide a marked contrast to the survival rates reported from clinical trials that largely enrol young male patients without significant comorbidity likely to complicate treatment and impact negatively on the patient's prognosis.[55]

Quality of life

Health related quality of life is being increasingly recognised as an important end point in trials of both pharmacological and non-pharmacological treatment strategies. Rather than solely measuring duration of survival, studies are being designed with a quality of life component in order to determine whether greater longevity equates to poor quality of life before an inevitable death. As the focus on the individual patient becomes more important, quality of life measures are even being incorporated into primary end points, rather than being measured as a secondary end point. This is particularly so when examining strategies where prolonging survival is not the principal concern.

Two large studies from the USA have shown that heart failure impairs self-reported quality of life more than any other common chronic medical disorder.[56,57] These findings have been confirmed by a recent European study.[58] Not surprisingly, quality of life deteriorates with increasing heart failure severity, and this is associated with increased numbers of physician visits, drug consumption, and hospitalisation. The prevalence of major depression in a hospitalised cohort of chronically ill patients aged over 60 years was found to be significantly greater in those with chronic heart failure (36·5% versus 25·5% for the remaining cohort). Depression is both prolonged and largely untreated in patients with chronic heart failure.[59,60] Dyspnoea, confusion and pain are also very common during the last few days of life in heart failure. The majority of patients would prefer "comfort care" and do not wish active resuscitation. Many would even prefer death.[60,61] It is not surprising, therefore, that there is a growing clamour for more attention to be paid to the end of life experience in

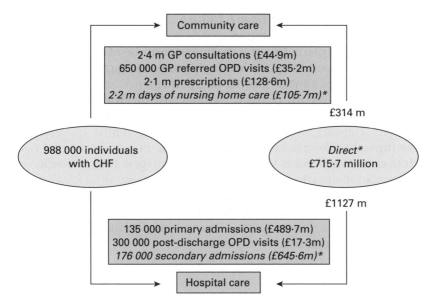

Figure 1.3   Cost of heart failure in UK (year 2000)

heart failure and the extension of palliative care services to improve the quality of life for a rising tide of such patients and their carers.[62,63]

Current impact of heart failure

As noted earlier, it is possible, using a combination of contemporary and reliable epidemiological parameters, healthcare utilisation rates and data relating to healthcare costs to estimate the overall burden and cost of heart failure within a whole country. Such an analysis was recently undertaken in relation to the UK population (approximately 60 million) and its health care system – the UK National Health Service.[49]

Figure 1.3 summarises the finding of this study providing a "snap-shot" of heart failure in the UK in the year 2000. It shows that apart from around one million individuals with symptomatic heart failure, in that country there were approximately 300 000 related hospitalisations, 2·4 million visits to general practitioners and over two million prescriptions. As described earlier, the overall cost of heart failure (including all related hospitalisations and nursing home care) in the year 2000 was approximately 4% of National Health Service expenditure.[49] As such, there is little reason to suggest that the experience of heart failure in other developed countries is any different.

The future direction of heart failure

Attempting to predict the future burden imposed by heart failure is fraught with uncertainty. For example contemporary estimates have predicted an exponential growth in the incidence and prevalence of heart failure when confronted with improved survival rates associated with acute coronary syndromes, sustained levels of hypertension, and the overall ageing of developed countries.[64,65] Whilst these studies have proved to be accurate in predicting the development of a heart failure epidemic there is some evidence to suggest that this epidemic will be sustained rather than increase dramatically.

Any examination of the future direction of the heart failure epidemic has to firstly focus on three specific ingredients:

- significant precursors
- rate of new/incident cases
- survival rates.

The first of these will determine whether the mixture of "fuels" that feed the current heart failure epidemic is likely to increase, decrease, or simply be sustained (for example the latter may occur if one "fuel source" is replaced by another). The second is a direct measure of how many new cases of heart failure are appearing per head of population (preferably this is described on a sex and age-specific basis). Any indication of the direction (either up or down) in the number of new cases will obviously be informative when considered in relation to the factors that will determine its future development. The last specific factor relates to average survival associated with heart failure. As noted above, the prognostic impact of heart failure is extremely high. Importantly, however, if we become better at prolonging heart failure related survival it is possible that the prevalence of heart failure will remain high even if incidence rates fall – remembering that the prevalence of heart failure (number affected at any one time) reflects the product of incidence times the average life expectancy of those affected.

The last more generalised but more predictable factor relates to the demographic profile of the population affected by heart failure. For example we do know that the average age of those affected by this syndrome is getting progressively higher.[55] What are the implications of this? Firstly, the older the individual with heart failure, the greater the associated morbidity (as reflected by visits to general practitioners and hospital stay); and secondly, older patients are much more complicated than younger individuals. In real terms, therefore, it might be possible for the overall prevalence of heart failure to fall, but the demand on the healthcare system to increase – a likely scenario given the ageing populations within developed countries.

Is the risk of developing heart failure falling?

It is important to note that although our understanding of heart failure continues to grow, there are still uncertainties about the relative contribution of the disease states commonly associated with this syndrome. For example coronary heart disease, either alone or in combination with hypertension, *seems* to be the commonest cause of heart failure. It is, however, very difficult to be certain what is the primary aetiology of heart failure in a patient with multiple potential causes (for example valvular disease in the presence of ischaemic heart disease and hypertension) and other common factors that have the potential to exacerbate underlying heart failure (for example atrial fibrillation and anaemia). Furthermore, even the absence of overt hypertension in a patient presenting with heart failure does not rule out an important aetiological role in the past, with normalisation of blood pressure as the patient develops pump failure. Data from both the Framingham[15,31] and Renfrew/Paisley studies,[66] which represent large-scale population cohorts followed up for a prolonged period, support the crucial role of hypertension in precipitating heart failure before acute manifestations of coronary heart disease emerge.

As indicated above, in the initial cohort of the Framingham Heart Study monitored until 1965, hypertension appeared to be the most common cause of heart failure, being identified as the primary cause in 30% of men and 20% of women and a co-factor in a further 33% and 25% cases respectively.[67] Furthermore, ECG evidence of left ventricular hypertrophy in the presence of hypertension carried an approximate 15-fold increased risk of developing heart failure. In the subsequent years of follow-up, however, coronary heart disease became increasingly prevalent prior to the development of heart failure and, as the identified cause of new cases of heart failure, increased from 22% in the 1950s to almost 70% in the 1970s. During this period, the relative contribution of hypertension and valvular heart disease declined dramatically. As such, there were approximately 5% and 30% declines in the prevalence per decade of hypertension during this period among men and women respectively.[68]

The apparent decline in the contribution of hypertension to heart failure most probably reflects the introduction of anti-hypertensive therapy; the parallel decline in the prevalence of left ventricular hypertrophy supports this supposition. In the latest data published by the Framingham investigators (see below) the declining role of hypertension in driving the incidence of heart failure in women was evident. Figure 1.4, showing data from the Olmsted County Study, clearly demonstrates that the incidence of heart failure following an acute myocardial infarction is declining – no doubt due to increased awareness of the importance of preserving ventricular function and integrity in the longer term.[69] On the other hand, despite a decline in

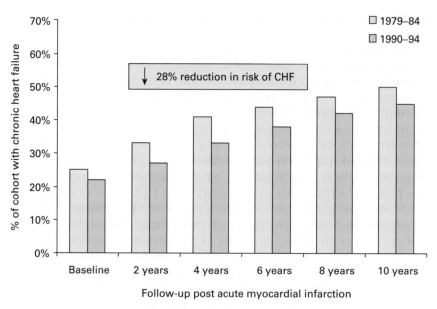

Figure 1.4 Falling incidence of heart failure post acute myocardial infarction in Olmsted County in the USA.[70] Adapted from original data

the number of cases of incident acute myocardial infarction (AMI),[70,71] parallel improvements in survival rates have the potential to "stabilise" the prevalence of "post-infarction" heart failure. Similarly, the continued presence of uncontrolled hypertension[72] within developed countries coupled with a rising epidemic of obesity[73] and diabetes associated with endothelial dysfunction[74] provides some indication that the potential for a substantive number of new cases of heart failure in the future is extremely high.

Declining incidence?

Unfortunately, much less is known about the incidence of heart failure compared with its prevalence. The most detailed incidence data emanates from the Framingham Heart Study.[75] After 34 years of follow-up of the Framingham cohort, the incidence rate was approximately 2 cases per 1000 in those aged 45–54 years, increasing to 40 cases per 1000 in men aged 85–94 years.[67,68] Using similar criteria, Eriksson and colleagues[17] reported incidence rates of "manifest" heart failure of 1·5, 4·3, and 10·2 cases per 1000, in men aged 50–54, 55–60, and 61–67 years respectively. More recently, Rodeheffer and colleagues[9] also reported the incidence of heart failure in a US population residing in Rochester during 1981 in persons aged

0–74 years. The annual incidence was 1·1 cases per 1000. Once again the incidence was higher in men than in women (1·57 versus 0·71 cases per 1000). It also increased with age – new cases increasing from 0.76 male cases per 1000 in those aged 45–49 years to 1·6 male cases per 1000 in those aged 65–69 years.

Cowie and colleagues reported an incidence study from a district of London with a population of approximately 150 000. In a 15-month period, 122 patients were referred to a special heart failure clinic, representing an annual referral rate of 6·5 cases per 1000 population. Using a broad definition of heart failure, only 29% of these patients were clearly diagnosed as having heart failure (annual incidence 1·85 per 1000 population).[76]

The critical question, of course, is whether the incidence of heart failure is increasing or declining? As described above, there is already some evidence to suggest that the rate of post-myocardial infarction heart failure in the USA is declining[69] and there is good evidence from several European countries that the rate of new hospitalisations for heart failure has stabilised since the mid-1990s.[41,42,44] Most strikingly, perhaps, are the data emanating from the most recent report from the Framingham Study[77] that show that the incidence of heart failure in this cohort has declined from 627 and 420 cases per 100 000 person years of follow-up in 1950–59 to 564 and 327 cases per 100 000 person years of follow-up in 1990–99, in men and women respectively: a decline of 7% and 31% in the risk of developing heart failure.[77] It is worth noting, however, that incidence rates for heart failure reached their lowest in 1980–89 in this cohort and the confidence intervals associated with these figures still provide some possibility that only a minimal decline in its incidence has taken place.

Improved survival?

There is increasing evidence from population based studies that the prognosis of heart failure (as described above) is beginning to improve with the introduction of more effective treatment modalities.[78] For example a seminal study of 66 547 Scottish patients admitted for the first time with heart failure during 1986–95 examined trends in short to longer-term survival rates in this cohort. Significantly, the median age at admission was 78 years in women and 72 years in men.[78] Just over half (53%) of this cohort was aged over 75. Consistent with the Rochester Study,[32] the median age of women (76·0 years in 1986 compared to 79·0 years in 1995) and men (70·7 years in 1986 compared to 73·0 years in 1995) increased significantly over the period of study (P < 0·001).

During the whole period of the Scottish study the crude case fatality rate at 30 days, 1, 5, and 10 years in men was 19·4%, 44·0%, 75·0%, and 87·2%, respectively. The equivalent rates were 20·3%, 44·9%,

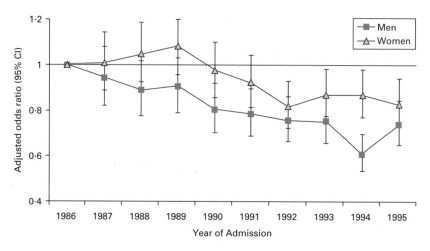

Figure 1.5 Reduced risk of all-cause mortality following an incident admission for heart failure in Scotland (1986–95).[79] Adapted from original data

76·2%, and 89·3% in women, respectively. Not surprisingly, case fatality rates increased markedly with age with one-month and one-year case fatality rates increasing from 10·4% and 24·2% in those aged < 55 years to 25·9% and 58·1% in those aged > 84 years. Median survival over the period of study was 1·5 years in men and 1·4 years in women. For those surviving the initial 30-day period, median survival was 2·5 years in men and 2·4 years in women.[78]

Figure 1.5 shows that, on an adjusted basis, the risk of case fatality in those admitted to a Scottish hospital with an incident case of heart failure in 1995 as compared to the 1986 cohort fell by 15% and 18% in men and women respectively.[78] Similarly, Figure 1.6, showing data from the Framingham cohort, shows that the risk of mortality in those who develop heart failure has progressively fallen from 1950 to 1999.[78] These recently published data have been supported by recent data emanating from Sweden.[44]

Projected burden of heart failure

Given the complicated messages imparted by indications that the common precursors of heart failure are under some control but some new precursors (for example obesity[73]) are not, trends indicating falling incidence rates, and what appears to be more prolonged survival associated with heart failure, predicting the future is fraught with uncertainty. However, the progressive ageing of the population (i.e. substantially more people at risk of developing heart disease,

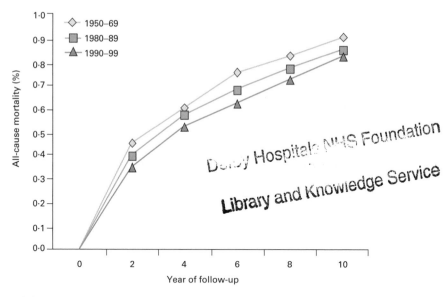

Figure 1.6 Improved survival rates in successive Framingham cohorts with clinically defined heart failure (1950–99).[78] Adapted from original data

hypertension, and then heart failure)[79] is a known factor that is likely to predicate a major change in the underlying prevalence of heart failure and produce a sustained epidemic.

Based on recent trends demonstrating that the heart failure epidemic has indeed stabilised but will likely be magnified by the ageing of the population, Figure 1.7 shows the most recent study predicting the likely profile of heart failure in a developed country – once again Scotland, where detailed epidemiological and demographic data are readily available.[80] As such, this figure shows that the most likely scenario is a gradual but not overly dramatic increase in heart failure related prevalence and healthcare activity over the next decade and beyond. Overall, it is projected that the number of men and women affected by heart failure will increase by 31% and 17% respectively with 52% more male and 16% more female incident admissions, respectively.[80] Certainly, these figures are far less dramatic than previously predicted[64,65] and the prediction that more men than women will be affected is markedly different from the current profile of heart failure.

There is little doubt, therefore, that the doubling in heart failure related costs in the UK during the period 1990–2000[63] will not be an isolated event – particularly given the prediction of increasing heart failure related hospitalisations. As the experience of heart failure has been remarkably similar in all developed countries there is also little

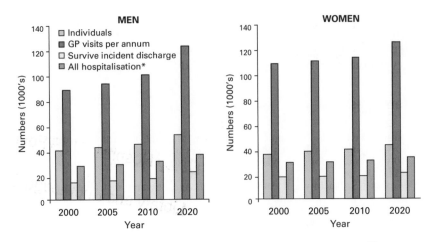

Figure 1.7 Predicted burden of heart failure in Scotland (2000–2020)[81]

doubt that the "international" cost of heart failure will also continue to rise without substantial changes in its prevention and treatment.

Conclusion

Chronic heart failure represents a growing health problem. Currently available pharmacological treatment strategies do not completely ameliorate the high morbidity and mortality rates associated with this truly malignant syndrome – especially in older individuals.[55] There is a clear need to develop and implement cost-effective programmes that prevent the development of heart failure (for example primary prevention in coronary heart disease). There is some hope that screening with markers such as brain natriuretic peptide[81] and rapid access echocardiography[82] may facilitate the process of detecting and treating individuals who still develop heart failure, as early as possible. However, a new "panacea" in screening and detection is unlikely given the heterogeneous nature of heart failure and the large number of individuals involved.

Unfortunately, therefore, the most urgent need relates to the increasing number of older individuals with chronic heart failure who are being hospitalised. Such individuals have limited survival prospects and are likely to have an extremely poor quality of life and require recurrent hospitalisation before they die.[48] It is within this context that specialist nurse intervention programmes have the potential to alleviate the overall burden of chronic heart failure by limiting costly hospital admissions, in addition to improving quality of life on an individual basis by providing more tailored and attentive health care. A large portion of this book is based on personal experience in developing and successfully applying this type of intervention in both the Northern[83] and Southern hemispheres.[84]

References

1 Tunstall-Pedoe H, Kuulasmaa K, Mahonen M, *et al.* Contribution of trends in survival and coronary-event rates to changes in coronary heart disease mortality: 10-year results from 37 WHO MONICA project populations. *Lancet* 1999;**353**: 1547–57.

2 Capewell S, MacIntyre K, Stewart S, *et al.* Age, sex and social trends in out-of-hospital cardiac deaths in Scotland 1986–95: a retrospective cohort study. *Lancet* 2001;**358**:1213–7.

3 McMurray JJV, Stewart S. The burden of heart failure. *Eur Heart J* 2003;**5**(Suppl I): I3–I13.

4 Task force for the Diagnosis and Treatment of Chronic Heart Failure, European Society of Cardiology, Remme WJ, Swedberg K. Guidelines for the diagnosis and treatment of chronic heart failure. *Eur Heart J* 2001;**22**:1527–60.

5 Logon WPD, Cushion AA. *Morbidity statistics from general practice*, vol. 1. Studies on Medical and Population Subjects No. 14. London: HMSO, 1958.

6 Gibson TC, White KL, Klainer LM. The prevalence of congestive heart failure in two rural communities. *J Chron Dis* 1966;**19**:141–52.

7 Royal College of General Practitioners, Office of Population Censuses and Surveys, and Department of Health and Social Security. *Morbidity statistics from general practice: third national study, 1981–82*. London: HMSO, 1988.

8 Parameshwar J, Shackell MM, Richardson A, Poole-Wilson PA, Sutton GC. Prevalence of heart failure in three general practices in north west London. *Br J Gen Pract* 1992;**42**:287–9.

9 Rodeheffer RJ, Jacobsen SJ, Gersh BJ, *et al.* The incidence and prevalence of congestive heart failure in Rochester, Minnesota. *Mayo Clin Proc* 1993;**68**:1143–50.

10 Mair FS, Crowley TS, Bundred PE. Prevalence, aetiology and management of heart failure in general practice. *Br J Gen Pract* 1996;**46**:77–9.

11 Royal College of General Practitioners, Office of Population Censuses and Surveys, and Department of Health and Social Security. *Morbidity statistics from general practice: fourth national study, 1991–92*. London: HMSO, 1995.

12 Clarke KW, Gray D, Hampton JR. How common is heart failure? Evidence from PACT (prescribing analysis and cost) data in Nottingham. *J Public Health Med* 1995; **17**:459–64.

13 Droller H, Pemberton J. Cardiovascular disease in a random sample of elderly people. *Br Heart J* 1953;**15**:199–204.

14 Garrison GE, McDonough JR, Hames CG, Stulb SC. Prevalence of chronic congestive heart failure in the population of Evans County, Georgia. *Am J Epidemiol* 1966;**83**:338–44.

15 McKee PA, Castelli WP, McNamara PM, Kannel WB. The natural history of congestive heart failure: the Framingham study. *N Engl J Med* 1971;**285**:1441–6.

16 Landahl S, Svanborg A, Astrand K. Heart volume and the prevalence of certain common cardiovascular disorders at 70 and 75 years of age. *Eur Heart J* 1984;**5**:326–31.

17 Eriksson H, Svardsudd K, Larsson B, *et al.* Risk factors for heart failure in the general population: the study of men born in 1913. *Eur Heart J* 1989;**10**:647–56.

18 Schocken DD, Arrieta MI, Leaverton PE, Ross EA. Prevalence and mortality rate of congestive heart failure in the United States. *J Am Coll Cardiol* 1992;**20**:301–6.

19 McDonagh TA, Morrison CE, Lawrence A, *et al.* Symptomatic and asymptomatic left-ventricular systolic dysfunction in an urban population. *Lancet* 1997;**350**: 829–33.

20 Davies MK, Hobbs FDR, Davis RC, *et al.* Prevalence of left ventricular systolic dysfunction and heart failure in the Echocardiographic Heart of England Screening study: a population based study. *Lancet* 2001;**358**:439–44.

21 Morgan S, Smith H, Simpson I, *et al*. Prevalence and clinical characteristics of left ventricular dysfunction among elderly patients in general practice setting: cross sectional survey. *BMJ* 1999;**318**:368–72.

22 Mosterd A, Hoes AW, de Bruyne MC, *et al*. Prevalence of heart failure and left ventricular dysfunction in the general population: the Rotterdam Study. *Eur Heart J* 1999;**20**:447–55.

23 Hedberg P, Lonnberg I, Jonason T, *et al*. Left ventricular systolic dysfunction in 75-year-old men and women: a population based study. *Eur Heart J* 2001;**22**:676–83.

24 Schunkert H, Broeckel U, Hense HW, Keil U, Riegger GA. Left ventricular dysfunction. *Lancet* 1998;**351**:372.

25 Gardin JM, Siscovick D, Anton-Culver H, *et al*. Sex, age and disease affect echocardiographic left ventricular mass and systolic function in the free-living elderly. The Cardiovascular Health Study. *Circulation* 1995;**91**:1739–48.

26 Kupari M, Lindroos M, Iivanainen AM, Heikkila J, Tilvis R. Congestive heart failure in old age: prevalence, mechanisms and 4-year prognosis in the Helsinki Ageing Study. *J Intern Med* 1997;**241**:387–94.

27 Devereux RB, Roman MJ, Paranicas M, *et al*. A population based assessment of left ventricular systolic dysfunction in middle-aged and older adults: the Strong Heart Study. *Am Heart J* 2001;**141**:439–46.

28 Nielsen OW, Hilden J, Larsen CT, Hansen JF. Cross sectional study estimating prevalence of heart failure and left ventricular systolic dysfunction in community patients at risk. *Heart* 2001;**86**:172–8.

29 Cortina A, Reguero J, Segovia E, *et al*. Prevalence of heart failure in Asturias (a region in the north of Spain). *Am J Cardiol* 2001;**87**:1417–9.

30 Kitzman DW, Gardin JM, Gottdiener JS, *et al*. Importance of heart failure with preserved systolic function in patients > or = 65 years of age. CHS Research Group. Cardiovascular Health Study. *Am J Cardiol* 2001;**87**:413–9.

31 Vasan RS, Larson MG, Benjamin EJ, Evans JC, Reiss CK, Levy D. Congestive heart failure in subjects with normal versus reduced left ventricular ejection fraction: prevalence and mortality in a population-based cohort. *J Am Coll Cardiol*. 1999;**33**:1948–55.

32 Senni M, Tribouilloy CM, Rodeheffer RJ, *et al*. Congestive heart failure in the community – Trends in incidence and survival in a 10-year period. *Arch Intern Med* 1999;**159**:29–34.

33 Ceia F, Fonseca C, Mota T, *et al*. Prevalence of chronic heart failure in Southwestern Europe: the EPICA Study. *Eur J Heart Fail* 2002;**4**:531–9.

34 McMurray J, McDonagh T, Morrison CE, Dargie HJ. Trends in hospitalization for heart failure in Scotland 1980–1990. *Eur Heart J* 1993;**14**:1158–62.

35 Rodriguez-Artalejo F, Guallar-Castillon P, Banegas Banegas JR, del Rey Calero J. Trends in hospitalization and mortality for heart failure in Spain, 1980–1993. *Eur Heart J* 1997;**18**:1771–9.

36 Ghali JK, Cooper R, Ford E. Trends in hospitalization rates for heart failure in the United States 1973–1986: evidence for screening population prevalence. *Arch Intern Med* 1992;**150**:769–73.

37 Haldeman GA, Croft JB, Giles WH, Rashidee A. Hospitalization of patients with heart failure: national hospital discharge survey 1985–1995. *Am Heart J* 1999;**137**: 352–60.

38 Eriksson H, Wilhelmsen L, Caidahl K, Svardsudd K. Epidemiology and prognosis of heart failure. *Z Kardiol* 1991;**80**:1–6.

39 Doughty R, Yee T, Sharpe N, *et al*. Hospital admissions and deaths due to congestive heart failure in New Zealand, 1988–91. *NZ Med J* 1995;**108**:473–5.

40 Reitsma JB, Mosterd A, de Craen AJM, *et al*. Increase in hospital admission rates for heart failure in the Netherlands, 1980–1993. *Heart* 1996;**76**:388–92.

41 Stewart S, MacIntyre K, MacLeod MMC, Bailey AEM, Capewell S, McMurray JJV. Trends in hospitalization for heart failure in Scotland, 1990–1996. An epidemic that has reached its peak? *Eur Heart J* 2001;**22**:209–17.

42 Mosterd A, Reitsma JB, Grobbee DE. Angiotensin converting enzyme inhibition and hospitalisation rates for heart failure in the Netherlands, 1980 to 1999: the end of an epidemic? *Heart* 2002;**87**:75–6.

43 Ng TP, Niti M. Trends and ethnic differences in hospital admissions and mortality for congestive heart failure in the elderly in Singapore, 1991 to 1998. *Heart* 2003;**89**:865–70.

44 Swedberg K, Köster M, Rosen M, *et al*. Decreasing one-year mortality from heart failure in Sweden: data from the Swedish Hospital Discharge Registry – 1988–2000. *J Am Coll Cardiol* 2002;**41**(suppl A):190A.

45 McMurray JJ, Hart W, Rhodes G. An evaluation of the cost of heart failure to the National Health Service in the UK. *Br J Med Econ* 1993;**6**:99–110.

46 Westert GP, Lagoe RJ, Keskimaki I, Leyland A, Murphy M. An international study of hospital readmissions and related utilization in Europe and the USA. *Health Policy* 2002;**61**:269–78.

47 Stewart S, Demers C, Murdoch DR, *et al*. Substantial between-hospital variation in outcome following first emergency admission for heart failure. *Eur Heart J* 2002; **23**:650–7.

48 McMurray JJ, Stewart S. Epidemiology, aetiology, and prognosis of heart failure. *Heart* 2000;**83**:596–602.

49 Stewart S, Jenkins A, Buchan S, McGuire A, Capewell S, McMurray JJ. The current cost of heart failure to the National Health Service in the UK. *Eur J Heart Fail* 2002;**4**:361–71.

50 Ho KK, Anderson KM, Kannel WB, *et al*. Survival after the onset of congestive heart failure in the Framingham Heart Study subjects. *Circulation* 1993;**88**:107–15.

51 Stewart S, MacIntyre K, Hole DJ, Capewell S, McMurray JJ. More 'malignant' than cancer? Five-year survival following a first admission for heart failure. *Eur J Heart Fail* 2001;**3**:315–22.

52 Peeters A, Mamun AA, Willekens F, Bonneux L. A cardiovascular life history. A life course analysis of the original Framingham Heart Study cohort. *Eur Heart J* 2002: **23**:458–66.

53 Jong P, Vowinckel E, Liu PP, Gong Y, Tu JV. Prognosis and determinants of survival in patients newly hospitalised for heart failure: a population based study. *Arch Intern Med* 2002;**162**:1689–94.

54 Cowie MR, Wood DA, Coats AJS, *et al*. Survival of patients with a new diagnosis of heart failure: a population based study. *Heart* 2001;**83**:505–10.

55 Petrie MC, Berry C, Stewart S, McMurray JJ. Failing ageing hearts. *Eur Heart J* 2001; **22**:1978–90.

56 Stewart AL, Greenfield S, Hays RD, *et al*. Functional status and well-being of patients with chronic conditions – results from the medical outcomes study. *JAMA* 1989;**262**:907–13.

57 Fryback DG, Dasbach EJ, Klein R, *et al*. The Beaver Dam Health Outcomes Study – initial catalog of health-state quality factors. *Med Dec Making* 1993;**13**:89–102.

58 Juenger J, Schellberg D, Kraemer S, *et al*. Health related quality of life in patients with congestive heart failure: comparison with other chronic diseases and relation to functional variables. *Heart* 2002;**87**:235–41.

59 Levenson JW, McCarthy EP, Lynn J, Davis RB, Phillips RS. The last six months of life for patients with congestive heart failure. *J Am Geriatr Soc* 2000;**48**:S101–9.

60 Krumholz HM, Phillips RS, Hamel MB, *et al*. Resuscitation preferences among patients with severe congestive heart failure: results from the SUPPORT project. *Circulation* 1998;**98**:648–55.

61 Koenig HG. Depression in hospitalized older patients with congestive heart failure. *Gen Hosp Psych* 1998; **20**: 29–43.

62 Murray SA, Boyd K, Kendall M, *et al*. Dying of lung cancer or cardiac failure: a community-based, prospective qualitative interview study of patients and their carers. *BMJ* 2002;**325**:929–33.

63 Stewart S, McMurray JJ. Palliative care for heart failure? *BMJ* 2002;**325**:915–6.

64 Kelly DT. Our future society: a global challenge. *Circulation* 1997;**95**:2459–64.

65 Bonneux L, Barendregt JJ, Meeter K, Bonsel GJ, van der Maas PJ. Estimating clinical morbidity due to ischemic heart disease and congestive heart failure: the future rise of heart failure. *Am J Publ Health* 1994;**84**:20–8.

66 Stewart S, Hart CL, Hole DJ, McMurray JJ. The incidence and natural history of heart failure in 15 406 men and women over 20 years: the Renfrew/Paisley Study. *Eur Heart J* 2001;**22**:208.

67 Kannel WB, Ho KK, Thom T. Changing epidemiological features of cardiac failure. *Br Heart J* 1994;**72**:S3–9.

68 Levy D, Larson MG, Vasan RS, Kannel WB, Ho KK. The progression from hypertension to congestive heart failure. *JAMA* 1996;**275**:1557–62.

69 Hellermann JP, Goraya TY, Jacobsen SJ, *et al.* Incidence of heart failure after myocardial infarction: is it changing over time? *Am J Epidemiol* 2003;**157**:1101–7.

70 Capewell S, Livingstone BM, MacIntyre K, *et al.* Trends in case-fatality in 117 718 patients admitted with acute myocardial infarction in Scotland. *Eur Heart J* 2001;**21**:1833–40.

71 MacIntyre K, Stewart S, Capewell S, *et al.* Heart of inequality – the relationship between socio-economic deprivation and death from a first acute myocardial infarction: a population-based analysis. *BMJ* 2001;**322**:1152–3.

72 Chobanian AV, Bakris GL, Black HR, *et al*; Joint National Committee on Prevention, Detection, Evaluation, and Treatment of High Blood Pressure. National Heart, Lung, and Blood Institute; National High Blood Pressure Education Program Coordinating Committee. Seventh Report of the Joint National Committee on Prevention, Detection, Evaluation, and Treatment of High Blood Pressure. *JAMA* 2003;**289**:2560–72.

73 Kenchaiah S, Evans JC, Levy D, *et al.* Obesity and the risk of heart failure. *N Engl J Med* 2002;**347**:305–13.

74 ACC/AHA Guidelines for the Evaluation and Management of Chronic Heart Failure in the Adult: Executive Summary: A Report of the American College of Cardiology/American Heart Association Task Force on Practice Guidelines (Committee to Revise the 1995 Guidelines for the Evaluation and Management of Heart Failure): Developed in Collaboration With the International Society for Heart and Lung Transplantation; Endorsed by the Heart Failure Society of America. *Circulation* 2001;**104**:2996–3007.

75 Margolis JR, Gillum RF, Feinleb M, Brasch RC, Fabsitz RR. Community surveillance for coronary heart disease: the Framingham Cardiovascular Disease Study. Methods and preliminary results. *Am J Epidemiol* 1974;**100**:425–36.

76 Cowie MR, Wood DA, Coats AJ, *et al.* Incidence and aetiology of heart failure: a population based study. *Eur Heart J* 1999;**20**:421–8.

77 Levy D, Kenchaiah S, Larson MG, *et al.* Long-term trends in the incidence of and survival with heart failure. *N Engl J Med* 2002;**347**:1397–402.

78 MacIntyre K, Capewell S, Stewart S, *et al.* Evidence of improving prognosis in heart failure: trends in case-fatality in 66 547 patients hospitalized between 1986 and 1995. *Circulation* 2000;**102**:1126–31.

79 Caselli G, Lopez AD. *Health and mortality among elderly populations.* New York: Clarendon Press, 1996.

80 Stewart S, MacIntyre K, Capewell S, McMurray JJ. Heart failure and the aging population: an increasing burden in the 21st century? *Heart* 2003;**89**:49–53.

81 Cowie MR, Struthers AD, Wood DA, *et al.* Value of natriuretic peptides in assessment of patients with possible new heart failure in primary care. *Lancet* 1997;**350**:1347–51.

82 Francis CM, Caruana L, Kearney P, *et al.* Open access echocardiography in management of heart failure in the community. *BMJ* 1995;**310**:634–6.

83 Blue L, Lang E, McMurray JJ, *et al.* Randomised controlled trial of specialist nurse intervention in heart failure. *BMJ* 2001;**323**:715–18.

84 Stewart S, Horowitz JD. Home-based intervention in congestive heart failure: long-term implications on readmission and survival. *Circulation* 2002;**105**:2861–6.

2: State of the art treatment for chronic heart failure

SIMON STEWART, JOHN MCMURRAY

Introduction

As described in Chapter 1, chronic heart failure is a heterogeneous syndrome whose impact can be measured in a number of different ways depending on the diagnostic criteria applied. The three most common forms of diagnostic criteria rely on clinical profile, objective measurement of cardiac function, or a combination of both.[1,2] This has made treating chronic heart failure on a uniform basis extremely problematic. The majority of large-scale clinical trials examining new treatment strategies for heart failure have focused on those individuals with moderate to severe left ventricular systolic dysfunction (i.e. a left ventricular ejection fraction < 40%). In the process they have tended to exclude women and older individuals.[3] The "real world" of heart failure management is, therefore, largely removed from the clinical trial experience.[4,5] Studies repeatedly demonstrate that prescribing patterns for heart failure rarely meet the standards demanded by contemporary guidelines.[6,7] This is also true of the level of diagnostic rigour used to determine the definitive presence and form of chronic heart failure being treated.[8] This last clinical issue is particularly relevant when considering the above mentioned evidence in support of the management of patients with chronic heart failure secondary to left ventricular systolic dysfunction as opposed to those who appear to have relatively preserved systolic function and possible left ventricular diastolic dysfunction.[9] Fortunately, there has been an increasing focus on determining the best form of treatment for this substantive group of patients.

It is within this context that this chapter briefly overviews the gold-standard treatment (both medical and surgical) of chronic heart failure associated with left ventricular systolic dysfunction with an update on the results and possible implications of recently completed studies. It also reviews the clinical implications of the recently reported CHARM studies in the management of the two most common forms of heart failure.[10–14] A more detailed description of the specific pharmacological agents and effective doses used in the management of heart failure are presented in Chapter 9.

Pharmacological treatment of heart failure

Diuretics

Although diuretics remain the cornerstone in managing the typical symptoms associated with sodium and water retention common to those with chronic heart failure, with the major exception of spironolactone[15] their definitive effect on survival has not been tested in long-term, randomised clinical trials. There is little possibility that the overwhelming anecdotal evidence in favour of diuretics, in addition to the availability of cheap generic brands, will permit a placebo-controlled randomised study of this class of agent in the future. There are, however, likely to be more trials that either examine the adjunctive impact of two different forms of diuretic (for example the Randomised Aldactone Evaluation Study, RALES[15]) or replace existing diuretic therapy with another form.[16–18]

It is important to note, that although diuretics relieve symptoms associated with sodium and water retention, they also have the potential to trigger neurohormonal activation in patients with mild heart failure. For example, the SOLVD treatment trial[19] showed that activation of the renin–angiotensin–aldosterone system was potentiated in those patients commenced on diuretics. Thus, diuretics should not be used as monotherapy for patients with heart failure.

Loop diuretics (most commonly furosemide) are most frequently used because of their ability to induce diuresis and therefore reduce the symptoms of congestion by reducing preload.[20] Moreover, loop diuretics are less likely than thiazides to precipitate worsening renal dysfunction when co-prescribed with an ACE inhibitor.[21,22] Overall, diuretics are commonly associated with symptomatic improvement and have been reported to reduce frequency of hospitalisation.[23,24] The specific adjunctive role of spironolactone is discussed below.

Angiotensin converting enzyme (ACE) inhibitors

In conjunction with diuretic therapy, ACE inhibitors have formed the cornerstone of heart failure management for the past decade. These agents have been shown to ameliorate symptoms, improve exercise capacity and left ventricular function as well as prolong survival in the whole spectrum of patients with left ventricular systolic dysfunction. The evidence for applying ACE inhibitors, therefore, exists for all patients with left ventricular systolic dysfunction regardless of whether they experience dyspnoea at rest (equivalent to NYHA Class IV) or remain completely asymptomatic.[25–31]

The ACE inhibitors specifically target the increased renin–angiotensin–aldosterone system activity associated with heart failure.

This activity results in greater concentrations of angiotensin II and aldosterone and therefore increased preload and afterload via greater vasoconstriction and sodium and water retention.[32] By decreasing the production of angiotensin II and inhibiting bradykinin catabolism, ACE inhibitors are thought to have a number of beneficial effects including:

- decreased cardiac preload and afterload
- prevention of ventricular remodelling
- decreased catabolism of bradykinin
- improved endothelial function and reduced oxidative stress.[33]

In the context of severe congestive heart failure, the Cooperative North Scandinavian Enalapril Survival Study (CONSENSUS) trial was the first study to show that ACE inhibitors have the potential to improve survival with an approximate 50% reduction in the risk of mortality at both 6 and 12 months associated with this agent.[26] More recent data, representing 10-year follow-up of almost all the original cohort participating in the study, demonstrated that the beneficial effects of enalapril in respect to survival were maintained for several years and the overall survival time was prolonged by approximately 50%.[31] The results of the landmark CONSENSUS study have been repeated in a number of subsequent studies that have consistently shown that ACE inhibitors improve survival and reduce hospital use among patients with chronic, moderate to severe heart failure.

It is of clinical significance to note that the ATLAS study[28] suggested that a higher dose of lisinopril (up to 35 mg/day and therefore comparable to the level of ACE inhibition achieved in the above mentioned clinical trials) was associated with a reduced incidence of death plus all-cause hospitalisation, as well as reduced heart failure admissions. This was in comparison to low dose lisinopril (2·5–5 mg/day and therefore more comparable to the level of ACE inhibition typically used in clinical practice). It is also worth noting that while the different ACE inhibitors may have slightly different pharmacological properties, they are generally accepted as having the same so-called "class effect" and can be applied with equal effectiveness in the treatment of all stages of heart failure (from asymptomatic to end-stage if tolerated).

β-blockers

The most promising development in the management of heart failure in recent years (pending a prolonged critique of the impact of adjunctive spironolactone therapy in the management of severe heart failure[34] and, similarly, the likely impact of the recently reported CHARM programme[11–14]) has been the establishment of the therapeutic benefit of applying a β-blocker as an adjunct to background diuretic and ACE inhibitor therapy for mild to moderate heart failure. These agents have long held the interest of clinicians for their ability to inhibit sympathetic nervous system activation and theoretically combat the progression of heart failure. As such, the sympathetic nervous system can be activated earlier and more substantially than the renin–angiotensin–aldosterone system.[35] The extent of this maladaptive process is independently predictive of subsequent mortality,[36] and forms a strong rationale for interrupting it through the application of β-blockade.[37]

The first multicentre trials of β-blockers in heart failure (the Metoprolol in Dilated Cardiomyopathy trial[38] and the Cardiac Insufficiency Bisoprolol Study [CIBIS I][39]) suggested that these agents improved both left ventricular function and the clinical status of heart failure patients. Moreover they reduced the need for cardiac transplantation. Subsequent studies in both the USA[40] and Australia[41] demonstrated that carvedilol (a β-blocker with ancillary vasodilatory and anti-oxidant properties) was associated with reduced hospitalisation, improved left ventricular function, and probably survival among patients with mild to moderate heart failure. In this context, further studies, the Cardiac Insufficiency Bisoprolol Study (CIBIS II)[42] and the Metorpolol CR/XL Randomised Intervention Trial in Heart Failure (MERIT-HF),[43] have demonstrated not only the ability of other β-blockers to reduce morbidity and mortality in patients with mild to moderate heart failure, but also that such treatment is associated with lower healthcare costs.[44]

Recently the Carvedilol Prospective Randomized Cumulative Survival (COPERNICUS) study has demonstrated that adjunctive treatment of severe, chronic heart failure with carvedilol was associated with improved survival and reduced morbidity. During an average of 10·4 months follow-up, adjunctive treatment with carvedilol was associated a 35% survival benefit and a 24% decrease in the risk of death or hospitalisation relative to the placebo arm of the study.[45] Alternatively, the results of the prematurely halted BEST study that examined the impact of bucindolol (a "third generation" non-selective β-blocker with vasodilatory properties most probably due to α_1-blockade) in 2708 patients with moderate–severe heart failure showed no survival benefits associated with this agent.[46] Indeed, a subsequent report highlighted an "early hazard" (combination of more adverse effects, greater hospitalisation, and higher mortality) evident in those classified with more severe heart failure (NYHA IV) at baseline in this study.[47]

The issue of a "class effect" in relation to applying β-blocker therapy in heart failure has, not surprisingly, been much more contentious than that relating to ACE inhibitors. For example, the relative reductions in mortality observed with bisoprolol, metoprolol, and carvedilol in mild–moderate heart failure patients were reported to be 34%,[42] 34%,[43] and 65%,[40] respectively. These agents have different properties and at present it is uncertain whether the greater reduction in mortality observed in the US carvedilol trials[40] is a chance finding or whether clinically important differences between these agents do exist. Certainly, the recent results of the Carvedilol or Metroprolol European Trial (COMET) study, a head-to-head comparison of metoprolol versus carvedilol in patients with moderate–severe heart failure associated with left ventricular systolic dysfunction, have ignited this debate. In this study, 1518 patients were randomised to a target dose of metoprolol 50 mg twice daily as opposed to 1511 patients randomised to carvedilol 25 mg twice daily.[48] During a mean of 58 months follow-up there was no difference in the composite end point of mortality and all-cause admission (74% versus 76%: P = 0·122) but a significant reduction in all-cause mortality in favour of carvedilol (34% versus 40%: hazard ratio 0·83; P = 0·0017). There are a number of key points arising from this study that are still the subject of some debate.

- The relative benefits of carvedilol were confined to survival and not to hospitalisation (largely neutral).
- The absolute and proportional number of sudden deaths in the carvedilol group was lower (218 [14%] versus 262 [17%]).
- The absolute number of cardiovascular-related deaths in the carvedilol group was markedly lower (438 versus 534) although the number of patients undergoing cardiac transplantation (censored event) and dying from circulatory failure was not substantially different.
- The dose of metoprolol used in the positive MDC (target 100–150 mg daily[38]) and MERIT trial (200 mg metoprolol succinate[43]) were markedly different from the dosage of metoprolol available and subsequently selected in the COMET study.[48]
- No formal comparison of carvedilol versus bisoprolol has been undertaken.

Overall, the results of the COMET study suggest the ancillary properties of carvedilol provide increased survival (but not morbidity) benefits to patients with chronic heart failure secondary to left ventricular systolic dysfunction relative to metoprolol. However, whether this effect would be sustained against current formulations of metoprolol and bisoprolol used to treat heart failure is unknown.

Spironolactone

As noted earlier there has been increasing interest in the adjunctive role of different combinations of diuretic therapy in managing heart failure. The major recipient of this has been spironolactone. Although spironolactone promotes less diuresis than furosemide it is an aldosterone antagonist and has a number of potential advantages when combined with a loop diuretic such as furosemide:

- enhanced diuresis
- additional aldosterone inhibition above that of ACE inhibitors which do not fully suppress aldosterone production in the typical setting of an activated renin–angiotensin–aldosterone system[49,50]
- growth factor inhibition.[51,52]

On this basis of the potential value of spironolactone, a pilot study (the RALES study) examined the value of this agent among chronic heart failure patients with symptoms indicative of NYHA Class III–IV. This study demonstrated that active treatment with spironolactone was associated with an increase in both plasma renin activity and urinary aldosterone excretion in addition to a decrease in atrial natriuretic factor.[53] A subsequent controlled study examining the effect of adjunctive spironolactone therapy on survival among patients with severe chronic heart failure was terminated prematurely due to significant mortality benefits associated with study treatment: all-cause mortality at two years was reduced from 46% in the placebo group to 35% in the spironolactone group, an absolute risk reduction of 11%.[15] In addition, there were fewer hospital admissions, improved symptoms and no significant increase in the risk of hyperkalaemia. As a result, spironolactone has now become part of the standard pharmacological management of patients with severe chronic heart failure – although not without some controversy due to higher adverse effects (predominantly hyperkalaemia) and residual concerns in respect to gynaecomastia or breast pain in male patients (10% incidence in RALES) than first anticipated.[54]

Angiotensin receptor blockers

Whilst the current pharmacotherapeutics used in the management of heart failure have been shown to generally improve health outcomes among chronic heart failure patients, the overall limitations of their therapeutic effect, even in clinical trials, have resulted in a continual interest in the development and subsequent study of new therapeutic agents. One of the most prominent and potentially effective of these is the angiotensin II receptor antagonists – otherwise known as angiotensin receptor blockers. Interest in the therapeutic benefits of suppression of angiotensin II release in heart failure arose from the observation that angiotensin II levels increase after prolonged ACE inhibitor treatment, theoretically reducing their beneficial effects.[55,56] Angiotensin receptor antagonists block the renin–angiotensin system directly at the angiotensin II receptor level and thus may provide more complete blockade of the effects of angiotensin II.[11]

The Evaluation of Losartan in the Elderly (ELITE) trial[57] was the first trial to compare the effects of the angiotensin receptor blocker losartan with an ACE inhibitor (captopril) in patients with heart failure. There was no difference between the two agents with respect to the primary end point of renal dysfunction. Unexpectedly, losartan was associated with lower mortality compared to captopril (4.8% versus 8.7%: a 46% risk reduction). To further investigate these promising data, the ELITE II trial[58] was performed in order to prospectively determine whether losartan conferred significant survival benefits over captopril. Overall, there was no statistically significant difference between losartan and captopril with respect to total mortality.

Based on these subsequent results from an appropriately powered and dedicated study, it has been accepted that ACE inhibitors should remain the cornerstone of treatment for patients with heart failure, and angiotensin II antagonists be used for patients who are intolerant of ACE inhibitors, for example due to cough or angio-oedema. The results of the CHARM-Alternative trial which recently reported the effects of candersartan (target dose 32 mg once daily) versus placebo in 2028 patients with symptomatic heart failure and a left ventricular ejection fraction of ≤ 40% who were previously found to be intolerant of ACE inhibitors (and were therefore not receiving any) has cemented this supposition. In this cohort, ACE inhibitor related problems including cough (72%), symptomatic hypotension (13%), and renal dysfunction (12%) precluded such therapy. During median follow-up of 34 months, patients randomised to candersartan had fewer primary end points (cardiovascular death or hospital admission for chronic heartfailure – 33% versus 40%: a 23% unadjusted risk reduction overall; P = 0·0004) with each component being reduced. Overall, the candersartan was relatively well tolerated compared to placebo (figures in brackets) with 3·7% (0·9%), 6·1% (2·7%), and 1·9% (0·3%) of this cohort experiencing symptomatic hypotension, renal dysfunction, and hyperkalaemia requiring study drug withdrawal.[13]

A key question has focused on whether the combination of an ACE inhibitor and an angiotensin receptor blocker is more beneficial than an ACE inhibitor alone in the management of chronic heart failure. Several smaller trials suggested that such a combination would be well tolerated in this clinical setting.[59,60] The Val-HeFT study[61] was a large randomised, placebo-controlled trial to determine whether there were incremental benefits associated with the addition of the angiotensin II antagonist valsartan to standard therapy (including ACE inhibitors) in patients with heart failure (NYHA II–IV). Patients received either valsartan (n = 2511, force-titrated to 160 mg twice daily) or placebo (n = 2499) in addition to prescribed heart failure therapy including ACE inhibitors (93%) and in some cases β-blockers (35%). Overall, valsartan was associated with a 13% risk reduction in the co-primary endpoint of death or cardiovascular morbidity.[61] However, it was clear that the major advantage of valsartan was in reducing recurrent hospitalisation with minimal adjunctive impact on mortality.[61,62] There was some concern that triple therapy (ACE inhibition, β-blockade, and angiontensin receptor blockade) was associated with worse outcomes in the 1610 patients receiving such a combination. As a result, there was conjecture that clinical trials had reached the limit of therapeutic neurohormonal blockade in chronic heart failure.[63]

The recently published results of the CHARM-Added trial[13] where placebo or candersartan therapy was randomly added to ACE inhibition in 2548 patients participating in the CHARM-Overall programme[11] have largely addressed these two important issues. Firstly, when provided as adjunctive therapy, candersartan was associated with a 15% unadjusted reduction (38% versus 42% over 41 months follow-up: P = 0.011) in the risk of cardiovascular death or hospitalisation when compared to standard heart failure therapy (100% ACE inhibitor use). Moreover, close analysis of those patients receiving concurrent β-blocker therapy (n = 1413) with prolonged follow-up showed that patients receiving candersartan had fewer primary events – as did those receiving higher doses of ACE inhibitors.[13] Overall, candersartan added to ACE inhibition was relatively well tolerated with 24% versus 18% study drug withdrawals compared to placebo. Common adverse events requiring such withdrawal (placebo comparison) included symptomatic hypotension 4·5% (3·1%), renal dysfunction 7·8% (4·1%), and hyperkalaemia 3·4% (0·7%). Pending updated guidelines, it would appear that candersartan added to conventional therapy (particularly in those patients in whom brain natriuretic peptide concentrations are high, indicating sustained renin–angiotensin–aldosterone activity[64,65]) could provide a relatively small but clinically significant improvement in health outcomes in those heart failure patients with impaired systolic function.[13]

Digoxin

Digoxin has been extensively used in the management of chronic heart failure for a number of years on the basis of the following beneficial effects:

- modulation of neurohormonal activity[66] resulting in decreased serum norepinephrine concentration,[67,68] improved baroreceptor function[67], and an overall decrease in sympathetic activity[69]

- electrophysiological effects resulting in decreased A-V nodal conduction and control of the ventricular conduction rate in patients with atrial fibrillation[70,71]
- positive inotropic effects mediated via Na$^+$ K$^+$ – ATPase inhibition.[72]

Despite its traditional use in chronic heart failure (although not without controversy), a definitive controlled study of the effects of digoxin among patients with mild to moderate chronic heart failure, in sinus rhythm and receiving ACE inhibitors, was only recently completed in 1997. In this respect, the Digitalis Investigation Group (DIG) study demonstrated no effect on mortality.[73] However, digoxin was associated with reduced hospital use especially that primarily associated with heart failure, and appeared to convey the most benefit to patients with more severe chronic heart failure. In this respect, a number of studies[74,75] have demonstrated that digoxin appears to convey the most benefit to patients with more severe heart failure and is associated with poorer health outcomes if withdrawn suddenly. As such, digoxin differs from all of the other oral pharmacological agents with positive inotropic properties, such as amrinone, milrinone, enoximone, and xamoterol, that have been proven in controlled studies to increase mortality when used to treat chronic heart failure patients.[76]

Antiplatelet and anticoagulation

The close, long-term link between thromboembolism and heart failure is well established.[77] For example, one early report of patients with idiopathic dilated cardiomyopathy showed a cumulative incidence of 3·5 stroke events per 100 patient years.[78] A review of the studies of patients with heart failure in which separate data for those not receiving anticoagulation were available showed that the overall incidence of arterial thromboembolism ranged from 0·9 to 5·5 events per 100 patient years.[79] Patients with atrial fibrillation and heart failure in particular are at high risk of thromboembolic complications and warfarin therapy has been shown to decrease the subsequent risk of stroke.[80] Thus, warfarin should be strongly considered for all patients with heart failure and concurrent atrial fibrillation.

A major issue has been the role of antiplatelet/anticoagulation therapy in those patients with heart failure who remain in sinus rhythm. A recent large-scale trial comparing the effects of warfarin, aspirin, and placebo in such patients was stopped early because of recruitment problems.[81]

A further trial, the Warfarin/Aspirin in Heart Failure (WASH) study,[82] was designed as a pilot study to test the feasibility of conducting a larger trial comparing aspirin (300 mg daily) and warfarin (target INR 2·5) and no antithrombotic therapy in patients with heart failure. A total of 279 patients were randomised in 17 centres in the UK and three in the USA. After mean follow-up of 27 months there was no difference between the three treatment groups with regard to the combined primary end point of all-cause mortality, non-fatal myocardial infarction and non-fatal stroke. However, there was an excess of hospitalisations in the aspirin group. Recently there have been concerns of potential adverse interactions between aspirin and ACE inhibitors in patients with heart failure.[83] A yet to be reported clinical trial, the WATCH study, is currently under way comparing warfarin (target INR 2·53), aspirin (162·5 mg daily) and clopidogrel (75 mg daily) in patients with heart failure.

Novel pharmacological agents

Natriuretic peptides

Although much attention has been paid to the role of atrial (ANP) and brain (BNP) natriuretic peptides in determining the presence of underlying heart failure (these neurohormones are increasingly secreted in response to volume expansion and pressure overload in the failing heart[84]) they may also provide a novel way of treating it. For example, clinical studies have shown that intravenous exogenous BNP (nesiritide) results in vasodilatation, diuresis, and natriuresis and antagonism of the renin–angiotensin system.[85,86] Studies examining the definitive clinical role of nesiritide (particularly as a treatment for acute decompensatory heart failure) are currently being undertaken.

Vasopeptidase inhibitors

Omapatrilat, a novel, dual-action vasopeptidase inhibitor, inhibits both neutral endopeptidase and angiotensin converting enzyme. It therefore increases natriuretic peptide levels (see above) in addition to decreasing angiotensin II levels.[87,88] The IMPRESS trial[89] compared the effects of omapatrilat with lisinopril in 573 patients with chronic heart failure over a 24-week period. The results suggest that omapatrilat was superior to lisinopril in improving symptoms and mortality/morbidity in heart failure.[89] The results of the Omapatrilat Versus Enalapril Randomized Trial of Utility in Reducing Events (OVERTURE) study in which 5770 patients with moderate to severe heart failure (NYHA Class II–IV) were randomised to enalapril (10 mg bd) or omipatrilat (40 mg) demonstrated that this novel agent is effective but might be useful only in select groups of patients. As such, during 14-month follow-up, the co-primary end point of risk of death or hospitalisation for heart failure requiring intravenous treatment demonstrated that it was neither inferior nor superior to enalapril therapy. The omapatrilat group did have a 9% lower risk of cardiovascular death or hospitalisation (P = 0·024) with post hoc analysis suggesting the most benefit occurred in respect to reduced hospitalisations for heart failure.[90]

Anticytokine therapy

Two recently aborted trials (RENAISSANCE and RECOVER) have provided strong evidence that anticytokine therapy is unlikely to provide another avenue of treatment for heart failure.[91]

Endothelial receptor antagonists

Bosentan is a non-peptide competitive antagonist, which blocks the effects of both endothelin A and B receptors. The REACH-1 trial was a multicentre, placebo-controlled trial of bosentan in patients with severe (NYHA IIIb/IV) heart failure.[91] The trial involved 370 patients and the primary end point was a composite of symptoms and major events at six months. The trial was stopped early by the Data and Safety Monitoring Board because of concern regarding liver dysfunction.[91] Overall there was no difference between the bosentan and placebo groups with regard to the clinical composite end point and the likelihood of this class of agent making a dramatic impact on the management of heart failure in the near future is low.

Treating anaemia in heart failure

There has been increasing recognition that the prognosis in heart failure worsens in the presence of anaemia (i.e. it is an independent prognostic marker).[92,93] In both uncontrolled and controlled studies of patients with heart failure and concurrent anaemia, correction of the anaemia with erythropoietin with or without the addition of intravenous iron has been attempted. The correction of anaemia has been associated with a marked improvement in NYHA functional class, improved cardiac function, and a marked reduction in the need for hospitalisation. It is also associated with improved exercise capacity, peak exercise oxygen utilisation and quality of life. Serum creatinine, which often rises steadily before treatment, is concurrently stabilised with the correction of underlying anaemia.[94] As such, this is a area of enormous interest in heart failure. For example, a major study called the Studies of Anaemia in Heart Failure Trial (STAMINA HeFT) is currently randomising 250 patients with chronic heart failure to either subcutaneous darbepoetin or placebo to determine its effect on functional status. Other studies examining iron supplementation are also under way.[95]

Devices

As sudden death, non-fatal arrhythmias, and bundle branch blocks are common in heart patients there has been increasing interest in the application of devices to improve cardiac output and prevent sudden death due to ventricular arrhythmia. Overall trials involving Class I and III anti-arrhythmic therapy (with the exception of amiodarone) alone have proven to be extremely disappointing. Such data are exemplified by the negative results of the SWORD study involving d-sotalol.[96] The GESICA study[97] showed a reduction in overall mortality in favour of amiodarone compared with placebo while the Survival Trial of Antiarrhythmic Therapy in Congestive Heart Failure (CHF-STAT) did not.[98] Further trials are under way to clarify the role of amiodarone in patients with heart failure.

Although implantable cardiac defibrillators have an established role in the management of patients with life-threatening ventricular arrhythmias,[99] their role in the primary prevention of ventricular arrhythmias and sudden death in patients with heart failure is uncertain. The Sudden Cardiac Death in Heart Failure Trial will determine the effects of amiodarone and implantable cardiac defibrillators on total mortality in patients with heart failure and left ventricular systolic dysfunction but without a history of ventricular tachycardia or fibrillation.

Biventricular pacing, in order to provide better synchronisation of the cardiac cycle in heart failure, has been shown in preliminary studies (for example the MIRACLE study[100]) to provide clinical benefits and is the subject of appropriately powered, large-scale randomised studies (for example the CARE-HF and COMPANION studies) that are close to being reported at this time (late 2003).[101] Although it is difficult to even predict the gold standard treatment of heart failure in the year 2005 (i.e. a time frame in which evidence from these trials will be incorporated into management guidelines) it is quite clear that the overall management of heart failure will become increasingly complicated with many therapeutic options available to the clinician.

Summary

The pharmacological management of chronic heart failure continues to evolve. Whilst there has been a strong emphasis on treating patients with systolic dysfunction, the design of the CHARM-Overall programme[11] may stimulate greater interest in those patients with preserved systolic function – thereby expanding treatment options for a significant cohort of patients. The key challenge is to be able to stay abreast of each new development and recommended guidelines, and apply them on an individual basis. The remainder of this book is devoted to how the evidence derived from clinical trials can be best applied in the real world through specialist nurse intervention in heart failure.

References

1 Remme WJ, Swedberg K. Guidelines for the diagnosis and treatment of chronic heart failure. *Eur Heart J* 2001;**22**:1527–60.
2 ACC/AHA Guidelines for the Evaluation and Management of Chronic Heart Failure in the Adult: Executive Summary: A Report of the American College of Cardiology/American Heart Association Task Force on Practice Guidelines (Committee to Revise the 1995 Guidelines for the Evaluation and Management of Heart Failure): Developed in Collaboration With the International Society for Heart and Lung Transplantation; Endorsed by the Heart Failure Society of America. *Circulation* 2001;**104**:2996–3007.
3 Petrie MC, Berry C, Stewart S, McMurray JJ. Failing ageing hearts. *Eur Heart J* 2001; **22**:1978–90.
4 Redfield MM. Heart failure – an epidemic of uncertain proportions. *N Engl J Med* 2002;**347**:1442–4.
5 Masoudi FA, Havranek EP, Wolfe P. Most hospitalized older persons do not meet the enrollment criteria for clinical trials in heart failure. *Am Heart J* 2003;**146**:250–7.
6 McLaughlin TJ, Soumerari SB, Willison DJ, *et al.* Adherence to national guidelines for drug treatment of suspected acute myocardial infarction: evidence for under-treatment in women and the elderly. *Arch Intern Med* 1996;**156**:799–805.
7 McDermott M, Lee P, Mehta S, Gheorghiade M. Patterns of angiotensin-converting enzyme inhibitor prescriptions, educational interventions, and outcomes among hospitalized patients with heart failure. *Clin Cardiol* 1998;**21**:261–68.
8 Francis CM, Caruana L, Kearney P, *et al.* Open access echocardiography in management of heart failure in the community. *BMJ* 1995;**310**:634–6.
9 Vasan RS, Larson MG, Benjamin EJ, *et al.* Congestive heart failure in subjects with normal versus reduced left ventricular ejection fraction: prevalence and mortality in a population-based cohort. *J Am Coll Cardiol.* 1999;**33**:1948–55.
10 Swedberg K, Pfeffer M, Granger C, *et al.* Candersartan in heart failure – assessment of reduction in mortality and morbidity (CHARM): rationale and design. CHARM-Programme Investigators. *J Cardiac Fail* 1999;**5**:276–82.
11 Pfeffer MA, Swedberg K, Granger CB, *et al.* Effects of candersartan on mortality and morbidity in patients with chronic heart failure: the CHARM-Overall programme. *Lancet* 2003;**362**:759–66.
12 Yusuf S, Pfeffer MA, Swedberg K, *et al.* Effects of candersartan in patients with chronic heart failure and preserved left ventricular ejection fraction: the CHARM-Preserved Trial. *Lancet* 2003;**362**:777–81.
13 McMurray JJ, Ostergren J, Swedberg K, *et al.* Effects of candersartan in patients with chronic heart failure and reduced left ventricular systolic function treated with ACE inhibitor: the CHARM-Added Trial. *Lancet* 2003;**362**:767–71.
14 Granger CB, McMurray JJ, Yusuf S, *et al.* Effects of candersartan in patients with chronic heart failure and reduced left ventricular systolic function intolerant to ACE inhibitors: the CHARM-Alternative Trial. *Lancet* 2003;**362**:772–6.
15 Pitt B, Zannad F, Remme WJ, *et al.* The effects of spironolactone on morbidity and mortality in patients with severe heart failure. Randomized Aldactone Evaluation Study Investigators. *N Engl J Med* 1999;**341**:709–17.

16 Stroupe KT, Forthofer MM, Brater DC, Murray MD. Healthcare costs of patients with heart failure treated with torasemide or furosemide. *Pharmacoeconomics* 2000;**17**:429–40.

17 Licata G, Di Pasquale P, Parrinello G. Effects of high-dose furosemide and small-volume hypertonic saline solution infusion in comparison with a high dose of furosemide as bolus in refractory congestive heart failure: long-term effects. *Am Heart J* 2003;**145**:459–66.

18 Cleland J, Gillen G, Dargie J. The effects of furosemide and angiotensin-converting enzyme inhibitors and the combination on cardiac and renal hemodynamics in heart failure. *Eur Heart J* 1988;**9**:132–41.

19 The SOLVD Investigators. Effect of enalapril on survival in patients with reduced left ventricular ejection fractions and congestive heart failure. *N Eng J Med* 1991; **325**:293–302.

20 O'Connor C, Gattis W, Swedburg K. Current and novel pharmacological approaches in advanced heart failure. *Am Heart J* 1998;**135**(suppl):S249–63.

21 Dyckner T, Wester P. Salt and water balance in congestive heart failure. *Acta Med Scand* 1986;**707**(suppl):27–31.

22 Baker DW, Konstam MA, Bottoft M, Pitt B. Management of heart failure. I Pharmacological treatment. *JAMA* 1994;**272**:1361–6.

23 Williams J, Bristow M, Fowler M, *et al*. Guidelines for the evaluation and management of heart failure. Report of the American College of Cardiology/American Heart Association Task Force on Practice Guidelines (Committee on Evaluation and Management of Heart Failure). *J Am Coll Cardiol* 1995;**26**:1376–98.

24 Richardson A, Bayliss J, Scriven A, Parameshwar J, Poole-Wilson P, Sutton G. Double blind comparison of captopril alone against furosemide plus amiloride in mild heart failure. *Lancet* 1987;**2**:709–11.

25 The SOLVD Investigators. Effect of enalapril on mortality and the development of heart failure in asymptomatic patients with reduced left ventricular ejection fractions. *N Eng J Med* 1992;**327**:685–91.

26 The CONSENSUS Trial Study Group. Effects of enalapril on mortality in severe congestive heart failure: results of the Cooperative North Scandinavian Enalapril Survival Study (CONSENSUS). *N Engl J Med* 1987;**316**:1429–35.

27 Pfeffer MA, Braunwald E, Moye LA, *et al*. on behalf of the SAVE Investigators. Effect of captopril on mortality and morbidity in patients with left ventricular dysfunction after myocardial infarction. Results of the Survival and Ventricular Enlargement Trial. *N Eng J Med* 1992;**327**:669–77.

28 Packer M, Poole-Wilson PA, Armstrong PW, *et al*. Comparative effects of low and high doses of the angiotensin-converting enzyme inhibitor, lisinopril, on morbidity and mortality in chronic heart failure. ATLAS Study Group. *Circulation* 1999;**100**(23):2312–18.

29 The Acute Infarction Ramipril Efficacy (AIRE) Investigators. Effect of ramipril on mortality and morbidity of survivors of acute myocardial infarction with clinical evidence of heart failure. *Lancet* 1993;**342**:821–8.

30 Kober L, Torp-Pedersen C, Carlsen JE, *et al*. for the Trandolapril Cardiac Evaluation (TRACE) Study Group. A clinical trial of the angiotensin-converting-enzyme inhibitor trandolapril in patients with left ventricular dysfunction after myocardial infarction. *N Engl J Med* 1995;**333**:1670–6.

31 Swedberg K, Kjekshus J, Snapinn S, for the CONSENSUS Investigators. Long-term survival in severe heart failure in patients with enalapril. *Eur Heart J* 1999;**20**: 136–9.

32 Packer M. Pathophysiology of chronic heart failure. *Lancet* 1992;**340**:88–95.

33 Tewksbury D. Angiotensinogen: biochemistry and molecular biology. In: Laragh J, Brenner B, eds. *Hypertension: pathophysiology, diagnosis and management*. New York: Raven Press; 1990:1197–216.

34 McMurray J, Cohen-Solal A, Dietz R, *et al*. Practical recommendations for the use of ACE inhibitors, β-blockers and spironolactone in heart failure: putting guidelines into practice. *Eur J Heart Fail* 2001;**3**:495–502.

35 Francis GS, Cohn JN, Johnson G, Rector TS, Goldman S, Simon A. for the V-HeFT VA Cooperative Study Group. Plasma norepinephrine, plasma renin activity and

congestive heart failure. Relationship to survival and effects of therapy in V-HeFT II. *Circulation* 1993;**87**(Suppl VI):VI40–48.

36 Cohn JN, Levine B, Olivari MT. Plasma norepinephrine as a guide to prognosis in patients with congestive heart failure. *N Eng J Med* 1984;**311**:819–23.

37 Doughty RN, MacMahon S, Sharpe N. β-blockers in heart failure: promising or proved? *J Am Coll Cardiol* 1994;**23**:814–21.

38 Waagstein F, Bristow MR, Swedberg K, *et al*. Beneficial effects of metoprolol in idiopathic dilated cardiomyopathy. Metoprolol in Dilated Cardiomyopathy (MDC) Trial Study Group. *Lancet* 1993;**342**:144–6.

39 The CIBIS Investigators. A randomized trial of β-blockade in heart failure: The Cardiac Insufficiency Bisoprolol Study (CIBIS). *Circulation* 1994;**90**:1765–73.

40 Packer M, Bristow MR, Cohn JN, *et al*. The effect of carvedilol on morbidity and mortality in patients with chronic heart failure. US Carvedilol Heart Failure Study Group. *N Engl J Med* 1996;**334**:1349–55.

41 The Australia–New Zealand Heart Failure Research Collaborative Group. Effects of carvedilol, a vasodilator β-blocker, in patients with congestive heart failure due to ischemic heart disease. *Circulation* 1995;**92**:212–18.

42 CIBIS II Investigators. The Cardiac Insufficiency Bisoprolol Study II (CIBIS II): a randomised trial. *Lancet* 1999;**353**:91–3.

43 Merit-HF Study Group. Effect of metoprolol CR/XL in chronic heart failure: Metoprolol CR/XL Randomised Intervention Trial in Congestive Heart Failure (MERIT-HF). *Lancet* 1999;**353**:2001–7.

44 CIBIS-II Investigators and Health Economics Group. Reduced costs with bisoprolol treatment for heart failure: an economic analysis of the second Cardiac Insufficiency Bisoprolol Study (CIBIS-II). *Eur Heart J* 2001;**22**:1021–31

45 Packer M, Coats AJS, Fowler MB, *et al*; Carvedilol Prospective Randomized Cumulative Survival (COPERNICUS) Study Group. Effect of carvedilol on survival in severe chronic heart failure. *N Engl J Med* 2001;**344**:1651–8.

46 BEST Trial Investigators. A trial of the β-blocker bucindolol in patients with advanced chronic heart failure. *N Engl J Med* 2001;**344**:1659–67.

47 Anderson JL, Krause-Steinrauf H, Goldman S, *et al*; BEST Investigators. Failure of benefit and early hazard of bucindolol for Class IV heart failure. *J Card Fail* 2003;**9**:266–77.

48 Poole-Wilson PA, Swedberg K, Cleland JGF, *et al*. Comparison of carvedilol and metoprolol on clinical outcomes in patients with chronic heart failure in Carvedilol Or Metoprolol European Trial (COMET): randomised controlled trial. *Lancet* 2003;**362**:71–3.

49 Marayev V, Skvortsov A, Masenko V, Belenkov Y. Escape of ACE inhibitor effects on aldosterone during long-term treatment of congestive heart failure. *International Meeting on Heart Failure*. Amsterdam; April, 1995.

50 Straessen J, Lijnen P, Fagard R, Verschueren L, Amery A. Rise in plasma concentration of aldosterone during long-term angiotensin II suppression. *J Endocrinol* 1981;**91**:457–65.

51 Young M, Fullerton M, Dilley R, Funder J. Mineralocorticoids, hypertension and cardiac fibrosis. *J Clin Invest* 1994;**93**:2578.

52 Hall C, Hall O. Hypertension and hypersalimentation. I. Aldosterone hypertension. *Lab Invest* 1965;**14**:285.

53 The RALES Investigators. Effectiveness of spirinolactone added to an angiotensin-converting enzyme inhibitor and a loop-diuretic for severe chronic congestive heart failure. *Am J Cardiol* 1996;**78**:902–7.

54 Berry C, McMurray JJ. Life-threatening hyperkalemia during combined therapy with angiotensin-converting enzyme inhibitors and spironolactone. *Am J Med* 2001;**111**:587.

55 Urata H, Healy B, Stewart RW, *et al*. Angiotensin II-forming pathways in normal and failing human hearts. *Circ Res* 1990;**66**:883–90.

56 Wolny A, Clozel JP, Rein J, *et al*. Functional and biochemical analysis of Angiotensin II-forming pathways in the human heart. *Circ Res* 1997;**80**:219–27.

57 Pitt B, Segal R, Martinez FA, *et al*. on behalf of the ELITE Study Investigators. Randomised trial of losartan versus captopril in patients over 65 with heart failure (Evaluation of Losartan in the Elderly Study, ELITE). *Lancet* 1997;**349**:747–52.

58 Pitt B, Poole-Wilson PA, Segal R, et al. Effect of losartan compared with captopril on mortality in patients with symptomatic heart failure: randomised trial – the Losartan Heart Failure Survival Study ELITE II. *Lancet* 2000;**355**: 1582–7.

59 McKelvie R, Yusuf S, Perjak D, Held P. Comparison of candersartan, enalapril and their combination in congestive heart failure: randomised evaluation of strategies for left ventricular dysfunction (RESOLVD Pilot Study). *Euro Heart J* 1998; **19**:133.

60 Hamroff G, Katz SD, Mancini D, et al. Addition of angiotensin II receptor blockade to maximal angiotensin-converting enzyme inhibition improves exercise capacity in patients with severe congestive heart failure. *Circulation* 1999; **99**:990–2.

61 Cohn JN, Tognoni G, Glazer RD, Spormann D, Hester A. Rationale and design of the Valsartan Heart Failure Trial: a large multinational trial to assess the effects of valsartan, an angiotensin-receptor blocker, on morbidity and mortality in chronic congestive heart failure. *J Cardiac Failure* 1999;**5**:155–60.

62 Cohn JN, Tognoni. A randomised trial of the angiotensin-receptor blocker valsartan in chronic heart failure. *N Engl J Med* 2001;**345**:1667–75.

63 Mehra MR, Uber PA, Francis GS. Heart failure therapy at a crossroad: are there limits to the neurohormonal model? *J Am Coll Cardiol* 2003;**41**:1606–10.

64 Troughton RW, Frampton CM, Yandle TG, et al. Treatment of heart failure guided by plasma aminoterminal brain natriuretic peptide (N-BNP) concentrations. *Lancet* 2000;**355**:1126–30.

65 Berger R, Stanek B, Frey B, et al. B-type natriuretic peptides (BNP and PRO-BNP) predict longterm survival in patients with advanced heart failure treated with atenolol. *J Heart Lung Transplant* 2001;**20**:251.

66 Gheorghiade M, Fergurson D. Digoxin: a neurohormonal modulator in heart failure? *Circulation* 1991;**84**:2181–6.

67 van Veldhuisen DJ, Man in't Veld AJ, Dunselman P, et al. Double-blind placebo-controlled study of ibopamine and digoxin in patients with mild to moderate heart failure: results of the Dutch Ibopamine Multicentre Trial (DIMT). *J Am Coll Cardiol* 1993;**22**:1564–73.

68 Krum H, Bigger J, Goldsmith R, Packer M. Effect of long-term digoxin therapy on autonomic function in patients with chronic heart failure. *J Am Coll Cardiol* 1995;**25**:289–94.

69 Ferguson D, Berg W, Sanders J, Roach J, Kempf J, Kienzle M. Sympathoinhibitory responses to digitalis glycosides in heart failure patients: direct evidence from sympathetic neural recordings. *Circulation* 1989;**80**:65–77.

70 Redfors A. The effect of different doses on subjective symptoms and physical working capacity in patients with atrial fibrillation. *Act Med Scand* 1971;**190**: 307–20.

71 Gold H, Cattel M, Greiner T, Catlove W, Benton J, Otto H. Clinical pharmacology of digoxin. *J Pharmacol Exp Ther* 1953;**109**:45–57.

72 Powell A, Horowitz J, Hasin Y, Syrjanen M, Horomidis S, Louis W. Acute myocardial uptake of digoxin in humans: correlations with hemodynamic and electrocardiographic effects. *J Am Coll Cardiol* 1990;**15**:1238–47.

73 The Digitalis Investigation Group. The effect of digoxin on mortality and morbidity in patients with heart failure. *N Engl J Med* 1997;**336**:525–33.

74 Uretsky BF, Young JB, Shahidi FE, et al. Randomized study assessing the effect of digoxin withdrawal in patients with mild to moderate chronic congestive heart failure: results of the PROVED trial. *J Am Coll Cardiol* 1993;**22**:955–62.

75 Packer M, Gheorghiade M, Young J, et al. Withdrawal of digoxin from patients with chronic heart failure treated with angiotensin-converting-enzyme inhibitors. RADIANCE Study. *N Engl J Med* 1993;**329**:1–7.

76 Reddy S, Benatar D, Gheorghiade M. Update on digoxin and other oral positive inotropic agents for chronic heart failure. *Curr Opin Cardiol* 1997;**12**:233–41.

77 Stewart S, Hart CL, Hole DA, McMurray JJV. A population-based study of the long term risks associated with atrial fibrillation: 20-year follow-up of the Renfrew/Paisley Study. *Am J Med* 2002;**113**:359–64.

78 Fuster V, Gersh BT, Giuliani ER, Tajik AJ, Brandenberg RO, Frye RL. The natural history of idiopathic dilated cardiomyopathy. *Am J Cardiol* 1981;**47**:525–31.

79 Baker DW, Wright RF. Management of heart failure. IV. Anticoagulation for patients with heart failure due to left ventricular systolic dysfunction. *JAMA* 1994;**272**:1614–18.

80 Stroke Prevention in Atrial Fibrillation Investigators. Stroke Prevention in Atrial Fibrillation Study: final results. *Circulation* 1991;**84**:527–39.

81 Cokkinos DV, Toutouzas PK. Antithrombotic therapy in heart failure: a randomized comparison of warfarin *v* aspirin (HELAS). *Eur J Heart Fail* 1999; **1**:419–23.

82 The WASH Study. Steering Committee Investigators. The WASH Study (Warfarin/ Aspirin in Heart Failure) rational design and end-points. *Eur J Heart Fail* 1999;**1**:95–9.

83 Cleland JGF. Anticoagulation and antiplatelet therapy in heart failure. *Curr Opin Cardiol* 1997;**12**:276–87.

84 Struthers AD. How to use natriuretic peptide levels for diagnosis and prognosis. *Eur Heart J* 1999;**20**:1374–5.

85 McGregor A, Richards M, Espiner E, Yandle T, Ikram H. Brain natriuretic peptide administration to man: actions and metabolism. *J Clin Endocrinol Metab* 1990; **70**:1103–7.

86 Holmes SJ, Espiner E, Richards AM, Yandle TG, Frampton C. Renal, endocrine and hemodynamic effects of human brain natriuretic peptide in normal man. *J Clin Endocrinol Metab* 1993;**76**:91–6.

87 Mills RM, LeJemtel TH, Horton DP, *et al.* on behalf of the Natrecor Study Group. Sustained hemodynamic effects of an infusion of nesiritide (human B-type natriuretic peptide) in heart failure: a randomized, double-blind, placebo-controlled clinical trial. *J Am Coll Cardiol* 1999;**34**:155–62.

88 Burnett JC. Vasopeptidase inhibition: a new concept in blood pressure management. *J Hypertension* 1999;**17**(suppl):S37–43.

89 Rouleau JL, Pfeffer MA, Stewart DJ, *et al.* Vasopeptidase inhibitor or angiotensin converting enzyme inhibitor in heart failure? Results of the IMPRESS Trial. *Circulation* 1999;**100**(Suppl 1):1–782.

90 Packer M, Califf RM, Konstam MA, *et al.* Comparison of omapatrilat and enalapril in patients with chronic heart failure: the Omapatrilat Versus Enalapril Randomized Trial of Utility in Reducing Events (OVERTURE). *Circulation* 2002;**106**:920–6.

91 Mylona P, Cleland JGF. Update of REACH-1 and MERIT-HF clinical trials in heart failure. *Eur J Heart Fail* 1999;**1**:197–200.

92 Kosiborod M, Smith GL, Radford MJ, *et al.* The prognostic importance of anemia in patients with heart failure. *Am J Med* 2003;**114**:112–9.

93 Szachniewicz J, Petruk-Kowalczyk J, Majda J, *et al.* Anaemia is an independent predictor of poor outcome in patients with chronic heart failure. *Int J Cardiol* 2003;**90**:303–8.

94 Silverberg DS, Wexler D, Blum M, *et al.* Erythropoietin should be part of congestive heart failure management. *Kidney Int Suppl* 2003;**87**:S40–7.

95 Mitka M. Researchers probe anemia – heart failure link. *JAMA* 2003;**290**:1835.

96 Waldo AL, Camm AJ, deRuyter H, *et al.* for the SWORD Investigators. Effect of d-sotalol on mortality in patients with left ventricular dysfunction after recent and remote myocardial infarction. *Lancet* 1996;**348**:7–12.

97 Doval HC, Nul DR, Grancelli HO, Perrone SV, Bortman GR, Curiel R. Randomised trial of low dose amiodarone in severe congestive heart failure. *Lancet* 1994;**344**:493–8.

98 Singh SN, Fletcher RD, Fisher SG, *et al.* Amiodarone in patients with congestive heart failure and asymptomatic ventricular arrhythmia. Survival Trial of Antiarrhythmic Therapy in Congestive Heart Failure. *N Engl J Med* 1995;**333**: 77–82.

99 Antiarrhythmics Versus Implantable Defibrillators Investigators. A comparison of antiarrhythmic drug therapy with implantable defibrillators in patients resuscitated from near-fatal ventricular arrhythmias. *N Engl J Med* 1997;**337**: 1576–83.

100 Louis A, Cleland JGF, Crabbe S, *et al*. Clinical trials update: CAPRICORN, COPERNICUS, MIRACLE, STAF, RITZ-2, RECOVER and RENAISSANCE and cachexia and cholesterol in heart failure. Highlights of the Scientific Sessions of the American College of Cardiology, 2001. *Eur J Heart Fail* 2001;**3**:381–7.

101 Cleland JGF, Coletta AP, Nikitin N, Louis A, Clark A. Update of clinical trials from the American College of Cardiology 2003; EPHESUS, SPORTIF-III, ASCOT, COMPANION, UK-Pace and T-Wave Alternans. *Eur J Heart Fail* 2003;**5**:391–8.

3: Specialist nurse intervention in chronic heart failure: the evidence to date

SIMON STEWART

Introduction

As discussed in Chapter 1, the overall burden imposed by an epidemic of heart failure in developed countries is both enormous and likely to be sustained in the immediate future. On an individual level, chronic heart failure confers extremely poor quality of life and the prospect of a premature death. To those closest to the patient with this syndrome the burden of care may be particularly difficult to bear. Moreover, healthcare systems, overall, fare little better in dealing with the problems and challenges imposed by heart failure.

Clearly, the range of effective treatment options outlined in Chapter 2 provides some hope for the future. However, merely prescribing the combination of a loop diuretic, a β-blocker, an angiotensin converting enzyme inhibitor and, perhaps, an angiotensin receptor blocker does not necessarily mean that the patient will either adhere to such a complex regimen or indeed tolerate it without experiencing significant adverse effects. Moreover, despite the combined benefits of such a regimen, as clearly demonstrated by well-designed clinical trials, there is no legitimate and widely available cure for heart failure and it remains a truly malignant syndrome.

It is within this context that there has been increasing interest in the role of specific heart failure management programmes, which involve a key role for the specialist heart failure nurse, to address unacceptably high morbidity and mortality rates and provide the type of care that the current healthcare system, regardless of its location, is unable to deliver. This chapter provides a critical overview of the current evidence (this remains an ever-expanding field of research) supporting the use of specialist nurse-led interventions in the management of heart failure following acute hospitalisation. In the past five years an increasing number of appropriately powered, randomised studies involving thousands of typically old and fragile patients with chronic heart failure have demonstrated that careful, individualised management, over and above gold-standard pharmacotherapy, is able to improve health outcomes in a cost-effective manner. Significantly, the effect of this type of intervention has been examined in sufficient numbers to warrant meta-analyses that confirm the type of benefits that the clinicians, who are so passionate in their delivery of such programmes of care, have no doubt exist. As such, this chapter provides clear evidence to support the type of programme described in detail in the later chapters of this book.

The individual burden of heart failure

In Chapter 1 the overall burden imposed by heart failure was examined in detail. Although the figures presented earlier might be of some interest to a clinician dealing with heart failure on a daily basis, there is little doubt the person affected by heart failure would be more reassured if the clinician paid greater attention to the day to day issues affecting the patient and their family. As noted, heart failure is not a homogeneous condition but rather a syndrome that is expressed in many different ways in individual patients – large-scale epidemiologically derived figures simply do not reflect this fact.

One of the first issues confronting the clinician dealing with heart failure at an individual level is the fact that the majority of patients bear little or no resemblance to those enrolled in clinical trials.[1,2] This is particularly true of those patients who experience an "acute crisis" and require some form of hospital treatment – an almost inevitable event when the "natural history" of heart failure (HF)[3,4] and the absence of a curative option for most patients[5] is considered.

These patients are typically of advanced age with concurrent disease states (typically chronic lung and renal disease) that both complicate the application of proven treatment strategies and increase their risk of subsequent morbidity and mortality.[6] For example, the role of concurrent anaemia in exacerbating heart failure has become the subject of intense interest and there is recognition that this condition has been a significant but largely overlooked factor in contributing to high levels of morbidity and mortality in many patients.[7] Such a contribution is not assisted by poor treatment and management strategies.[8] In such patients quality of life is usually extremely poor,[9] frequent admissions are the norm[10] (particularly in winter months[11,12]) and a premature death likely.[13-15] Without appropriate support, the burden of caring for someone with heart failure is immense and likely to severely impair the carer's quality of life.[16]

It is clear from the epidemiological/economic data described above that if it were possible to manage these typically older patients more effectively and replace costly hospitalisations with less expensive health care then substantial economic benefits would be derived – see Chapter 5. Sadly, it is probably economic rather than individual considerations that have generated an increasing interest in specific programmes designed to optimise the management of heart failure and produce better health outcomes (i.e. reduced hospital use). Fortunately, as described below, these programmes have had the positive "side effect" of improving the lives of many individual patients as well as delivering economic benefits.

Identifying barriers to better health outcomes in heart failure

Any attempt to minimise the impact of heart failure, due to its heterogeneity and the complex treatment and management issues it engenders, has to focus on inherent problems at the individual level. The apparent inability of many individuals with heart failure (remembering that a significant proportion of patients do improve with treatment) to gain the maximum clinical benefit from otherwise proven therapeutics is obviously a vexing problem. However, relatively poor outcomes should come as no surprise given the nature of the syndrome and the inherently complex interaction between the individual, their treatment, and the many components of the health-care system within which they are managed. Anything that interrupts or hinders what should be a harmonious and productive interaction between the patient and the healthcare system has the potential to lead to a lack of symptom control, unplanned hospitalisation, and even premature death (key features of the natural history of heart failure).

Whilst inherently "high risk" patients would benefit most from appropriate and consistent treatment they are, unfortunately, at greatest risk from those factors that commonly precipitate sub-optimal treatment of heart failure. Their frequent inability to tolerate even minor fluctuations in their cardiac, and commonly their renal, function leaves them vulnerable to frequent and recurrent episodes of acute heart failure. They are, therefore, at risk of both frequent hospitalisation for heart failure and other related conditions.

It is within this context that there are many preventable and often interrelated factors contributing to poorer outcomes among typically older patients with heart failure. These potentially modifiable factors can be summarised as follows:

- inadequate/inappropriate medical treatment or adverse effects of prescribed treatment
- inadequate knowledge of the underlying illness and prescribed treatment

- inadequate response to, or recognition of, acute episodes of clinical deterioration
- non-adherence to prescribed pharmacological treatment
- lack of motivation/inability to adhere to a non-pharmacological management plan
- problems with caregivers or extended care facilities
- poor social support.[17–22]

It is not surprising, therefore, that there are data to suggest that up to two thirds of heart failure related hospitalisations are preventable.[19–22,23] Many of the factors listed above are often addressed in the "usual care" arms of clinical trials, with the provision of increased monitoring and individualised follow-up. It is not surprising, therefore, that patients in clinical trials usually have lower than anticipated morbidity and mortality rates[1] and that the programmes described below have many similar features to those built into clinical trials.

Development of heart failure programmes of care: key issues and features

Before discussing the relative benefits of applying more effective programmes of health care specifically designed to optimise the management of heart failure, it is important to review five of the most important issues that have shaped the attempts thus far to improve heart failure related outcomes at both population and individual level.

1. It is clear that apart from preventing patients from developing heart failure (obviously established primary prevention strategies[24] and, more recently, the HOPE study[25] are relevant to this) the greatest cost benefits are likely to be derived from targeting patients with heart failure who have already been hospitalised – particularly old and fragile patients at high risk of subsequent morbidity and mortality.
2. It is important to recognise that whilst a proportion of heart failure related admissions are indeed avoidable, a similar proportion are likely to be either inevitable for adequate treatment of an acute clinical crisis or even desirable to provide for adequate investigation and future management.
3. Precipitating factors leading to a heart failure related admission are often multifactorial and interrelated. The typical profile of the older patient with heart failure who has been hospitalised (for example with acute decompensated heart failure secondary to uncontrolled atrial fibrillation and underlying anaemia) is often complex, and identifying contributory factors is often nebulous.

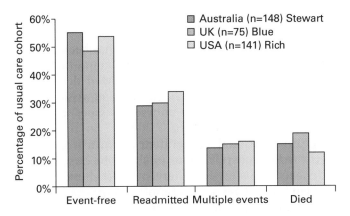

Figure 3.1 Comparison of 90-day outcomes in typically old and fragile patients with chronic heart failure exposed to usual care in Australia,[28] the UK,[29] and the USA[30]

4. Given the often extensive list of concurrent disease states in older patients with heart failure, it is frequently difficult to determine its exact role in precipitating acute events. As such, the proportion of hospitalisations that can be identified as directly attributable to the syndrome (even if frequent) is often less than 50%.

5. Regardless of the purpose of an intervention designed to limit heart failure related morbidity rates (and therefore costs) and the often overwhelming imperative to minimise the expense of a programme whilst maximising subsequent cost savings, it is important to appreciate the degree of comfort and satisfaction patients with heart failure derive from receiving individualised care and support.

Given the above, it should come as no surprise how the general body of research in this area has developed and the general direction it has taken. Firstly, most of the early studies (between 1995 and 2000) testing the relative benefits of programmes of care in heart failure targeted hospitalised patients and applied interventions during or immediately following their index admission.[26,27] Not surprisingly, those studies targeting typically older "high risk" patients have proven to be the most cost-effective when resulting in reduced hospital admissions and associated stay in the presence of high underlying morbidity and mortality rates. Figure 3.1, for example, shows the typically high (and consistent, despite the differences in healthcare delivery) event rates in the study cohorts of key studies undertaken in Australia,[28] the UK,[29] and the USA[30] where patients were randomly allocated to usual care.[31]

Studies to date have typically worked on the assumption that an approximate halving in recurrent hospitalisation in the short to medium term is feasible.[26,27] Although there has been a trend towards a more specific and exclusive focus on managing heart failure more effectively, the greatest cost benefits have been derived from those programmes of care that reduce "all-cause" readmissions (for example by focusing on general treatment adherence issues) rather than heart failure related readmissions alone.[27] Related to the cost dynamics of applying an additional component of health care in order to subsequently reduce costs,[32] there was an obvious need to apply a relatively "cheap" but effective intervention (i.e. one that reduces all-cause recurrent stay). Given the complex nature of heart failure and factors precipitating clinical instability[22] it was perhaps not surprising that one-dimensional interventions (for example providing pre-discharge education) have proved to be relatively ineffective and were quickly discarded in favour of flexible but individualised interventions delivered or coordinated (within a multidisciplinary context) by suitably trained nurses.

Over a relatively short period of time the role of the "specialist heart failure nurse" (or other derivatives) has expanded to maximise the time they can spend with the patient – most notably prescribing and titration of pharmacotherapy (for example angiotensin converting enzyme (ACE) inhibitors and β-blockers). Given the inherent satisfaction of heart failure patients with this type of contact (i.e. with a caring nurse), and the emergence of academic nurses as principal investigators of these studies, it should come as no surprise that spending time with patients on a individual basis has become an important feature of these programmes. In order to "protect" this individual time from future cost cutting measures, it will be important for specialist heart failure nurses to quantify the therapeutic benefits of such contact.

It is within this context that the number of post-discharge heart failure programmes of care involving a key role for the specialist heart failure nurse has exploded. A number of key features are common to nearly all these programmes:

- a multidisciplinary approach
- individualised care
- patient education and counselling (often involving the family/carer)
- intensive follow-up to detect and address clinical problems on a proactive basis
- strategies to both apply evidence-based pharmacological treatment and improve adherence
- application of non-pharmacological strategies where appropriate (for example fluid and electrolyte management and exercise programmes)
- patient-initiated access to appropriate advice and support.[26,27]

A major goal of this type of programme is to encourage a greater level of effective self-care behaviours in the majority of patients (for example daily weight monitoring, applying a diuretic regimen and recognising signs of acute heart failure and seeking appropriate health care) and only filling the "gaps" in certain cases (for example an older patient who lives alone).[33] Determining the most desirable and effective role of interactive technology that can provide a greater level of patient surveillance (for example via computerised tracking of a patient's clinical status using a home monitoring device) while encouraging a degree of independence from the healthcare system is probably yet to be achieved. Certainly, there is a growing body of research examining the role of "remote" health care. Striking the balance between providing therapeutic human contact, promoting self-care behaviours, and monitoring a patient's clinical status without creating a "Big Brother" scenario of excessive intrusion is a major challenge for the future.

Key studies of heart failure programmes of care

There now exists an increasing body of research to support the application of post-discharge heart failure programmes, with a major role for a specialist heart failure nurse in most cases – the one exception being a pharmacist-based intervention.[34] It is important to note, however, that a large number of published research studies have either involved a small number of patients, or have had limited follow-up, or have measured the influence of a particular programme using pre- and post-testing periods or historical control data.[35-47] While these studies are important to the general body of literature, it is most appropriate to examine the results of appropriately powered studies that employed a randomised design – particularly as other designs inherently inflate the observed magnitude of effect. Table 3.1 provides an overview of 18 of the largest randomised studies involving study follow-up of three months or longer with study cohorts limited to the hundreds rather than thousands due to the greater potential for clinically significant improvements in outcomes when including typically older heart failure patients.[29-31,34, 48-61] It is important to note that this table does not include a number of positive studies where heart failure was not the main focus of the published report (i.e. it included heterogeneous patients with a variety of chronic cardiac disease states[62-64]) or where the study is yet to be published as a full report.[65,66]

Notable studies

A number of the studies outlined in the table deserve special comment on the basis that they were appropriately powered

Table 3.1 Randomised controlled studies of post-discharge programmes designed to improve health outcomes in patients with heart failure[29-31,34,48-61]

Study	Study cohort	Study intervention	Major end points	Results	Comments
Strömberg, et al. Eur Heart J 2003 (Sweden)	**106** HF pts admitted to one academic and two county hospitals in Sweden.	Nurse-led heart failure clinic staffed by specialist heart failure nurses.	All-cause mortality or readmission at **12 months**.	Study patients had fewer primary end points (29 vs. 40: P = 0·03) and fewer deaths (7 vs. 20: P = 0·005). Study patients also had fewer days of hospital admission (350 vs. 592: P = 0·045). The intervention also improved self-care behaviours.	This study confirmed the potential impact of these programmes on survival in addition to cementing the role of nurse-led clinics.
Stewart, et al. Circulation 2002 (Australia)	Combined analysis of **298** "high risk" HF pts aged ≥ 55 years from a university hospital in Adelaide who were discharged to home and participated in the two previously reported studies.	Multidisciplinary, home-based intervention with post-discharge home visits at 7–14 days. The second study was more HF-specific than the first.	Frequency of unplanned readmissions plus out-of-hospital deaths during **3–6 years follow-up (median 4·2 years).**	Study patients had fewer primary events (mean of 0·21 vs. 0·37 events/pt/mth: P < 0·01). Median event-free (7 vs. 3 mths: P < 0·01) and all-cause survival (40 vs. 22 mths: P < 0·05) was also more prolonged.	This is the first study to examine the effect of this type of intervention beyond two years and provides preliminary evidence to suggest that it is possible to cost-effectively prolong survival and reduce hospital stay.
Kasper EK, et al. J Am Coll Cardiol 2002 (USA)	**200** "high risk" HF pts admitted to the Johns Hopkins Hospital & the Johns Hopkins Bayview Medical Center.	Multidisciplinary management programme with pre-specified schedule of contacts with a CHF nurse (mainly clinic visits) and telephone follow-up.	Death from any cause plus admissions for HF, all hospital admissions and quality of life within **6 months**.	The primary end point occurred less frequently in the study group compared to usual care (7 vs. 13 deaths and 43 vs. 59 admissions: P = 0·09). Overall, study pts had fewer days of readmission (4·3 vs. 6·3/pt: NS). Quality of life scores were significantly improved.	This was a relatively young cohort of CHF patients: possibly because patients with renal dysfunction were excluded – event rates were low as a result. The study intervention was similar to that employed in the study by Blue et al – but on a clinic basis – with less effect.

(Continued)

Table 3.1 continued

Study	Study cohort	Study intervention	Major end points	Results	Comments
Harrison, et al. Med Care 2002 (Canada)	157 (originally 192) HF pts admitted to two medical units in Ottawa, Ontario.	Transitional care model to improve patient education and level of usual home care.	Change in quality of life scores within 12 weeks.	Quality of life as measured by the Minnesota Living With Heart Failure Questionnaire was significantly improved in the study group. Study pts tended to have fewer admissions (NS).	This study concentrated almost exclusively on quality of life and showed improvements with the intervention – although it also improved in the usual care group.
Riegel, et al. Arch Intern Med 2002 (USA)	242 (originally 358) HF pts recruited from two southern Californian Hospitals. It is unclear if these were "high risk" patients – the majority of pts were in NYHA Class III/IV at hospital discharge.	Nurse-directed, telephonic case management programme (average of 17 phone calls over 6 months). Additional guidelines to physicians.	HF-related admissions and associated stay within 6 months.	Rate of HF-related admissions was reduced by 48% (P < 0·05) and associated stay by 46% (P < 0·05). However, all-cause stay was 28% less in the study group (NS). The cost of care also tended to be lower (NS).	A major feature of this study was the major loss to follow-up. It does represent the first large study of telephone follow-up and whilst HF-related outcomes improved, it was less effective overall (all-cause events: NS).
Krumholz, et al. J Am Coll Cardiol 2002 (USA)	88 HF pts aged > 50 years recruited from Yale–New Haven Hospital.	Educational programme covering 5 sequential care domains for self-care of chronic disease. 55%:45% clinic visits vs. home visits plus telephone follow-up.	Event-free survival, HF-related morbidity and all-cause deaths within 1 year.	Event-free survival was more prolonged in the study group (HR 0·56: P < 0·05). Fewer study pts readmitted for HF (57% vs. 82%: P = 0·01). Study pts tended to have fewer all-cause days of readmission/pt (10·2 vs. 15·2: P = 0·09).	Although described as uniquely focused on education alone the study has similarities to that performed by Jaarsma et al. Whether education "alone" was provided is debatable due to home/ clinic visits + telephone "advice".
Doughty, et al. Eur Heart J 2002 (New Zealand)	197 CHF patients admitted to a tertiary hospital in Auckland.	An integrated HF management programme with a combination of	Event-free survival, all-cause readmissions and stay and	There was no difference in event-free survival and more pts had a primary event (68 vs. 61: NS) in the study group. The rate	This was essentially a clinic-based intervention. Although the majority of results were disappointing,

(Continued)

Table 3.1 continued

Study	Study cohort	Study intervention	Major end points	Results	Comments
		clinic-based follow-up and primary care visits.	quality of life within **1 year**	of readmission was lower by 26% and fewer bed days (NS).	the study programme did reduce hospital stay overall.
Blue, et al. BMJ 2002 (United Kingdom)	**165** HF pts admitted to a tertiary referral hospital in Glasgow.	Nurse-led home-based programme of care with multiple home visits and initiation/titration of pharmacological therapy.	All-cause death and HF admission within **3–12 months**. HF and all-cause stay.	Pts in the study group were less likely to have a primary event (HR 0·61: P < 0·05). Study pts also had fewer all-cause readmissions (86 vs. 114: P < 0·05) and associated stay (P < 0·05).	This is the first randomised study to examine a programme of care where specialist nurses initiated and titrated pharma-cotherapy. Home visits were more frequent than Stewart et al.
McDonald, et al. Eur J Heart Fail 2001 (Ireland)	**98** CHF pts admitted to a tertiary referral hospital in Dublin.	Inpatient and outpatient education and close telephone and clinic follow-up added to gold-standard pharmacotherapy.	Event-free survival at **90 days** (HF readmission or death) and **1 month readmission**.	No readmissions at 1 month in both groups. At 3 months, 4 vs. 14 end points recorded in each group (P = 0·02).	This study had very low end points and remains an "outlier" in the reported literature – the authors believe gold-standard treatment is responsible for the results.
Stewart, et al. Lancet 1999 (Australia)	**200** HF pts aged ≥ 55 years recruited from a university hospital in Adelaide (South Australia).	Multidisciplinary, home-based intervention with at least one home visit by a cardiac nurse.	Frequency of unplanned readmissions plus out-of-hospital deaths within **6 months**.	Usual care patients had more (129 vs. 77) primary events (P = 0·02) and more study pts remained event-free (38 vs. 51; P = 0·04) at 6 months.	This is the first study to show that this type of intervention is associated with both prolonged event-free survival and fewer readmissions. It also suggested survival benefits.
Jaarsma, et al. Eur Heart J 1999 (Netherlands)	**179** HF pts from a university hospital.	A supportive education programme in the hospital and	Self-care behaviour and healthcare utilisation	The intervention increased self-care behaviour. There were strong associated trends	This singular strategy was beneficial overall, although none of the

(Continued)

Table 3.1 continued

Study	Study cohort	Study intervention	Major end points	Results	Comments
		home promoting self-care behaviour.	within **9 months**.	towards fewer pts readmitted and fewer days of admission.	healthcare utilisation end points reached statistical significance. It confirms the importance of pt education.
Stewart, et al. Arch Intern Med 1999 (Australia)	**97** HF pts admitted to a tertiary referral hospital in Adelaide, who participated in a larger study of a home intervention (n = 762).	A combination of pre-discharge education and a home visit by a nurse and pharmacist.	Event-free survival and hospital readmissions within **18 months**.	Pts in the study group had fewer primary events (66 vs. 135 events: P < 0·05) and fewer days of hospitalisation (2·5 vs. 4·5/pt: P < 0·01).	This was the first study to suggest that this type of intervention had longer-term beneficial effects on both readmission and survival.
Oddone, et al. Eff Clin Pract 1999 (USA)	**433** male HF pts who participated in a larger randomised study (n = 1396) of increased accessed to primary care in 9 Veteran Affairs hospitals.	Increased access to primary care via a dedicated nurse and physician in addition to telephone and clinic follow-up.	Health-related quality of life and readmission rates.	No influence on quality of life. Increased rate of hospitalisation in the intervention group: a mean 1·5 vs. 1·1 readmissions per 6 months of follow-up (P = 0·02).	This is the only reported (a key point!) negative trial of this type of intervention. It largely revolved around a non-specific primary care intervention.
Gattis, et al. Arch Intern Med 1999 (USA)	**181** HF pts admitted to the Duke University Medical Centre with mild to moderate heart failure.	A pharmacist intervention to optimise the pharmacotherapy during the index admission plus telephone follow-up.	All cause mortality and heart failure clinical events within **6 months**.	Fewer primary events in the study group (4 vs. 16: P = 0·01). Evidence-based treatment was greater in the study group.	Event rates were very low in the study cohort – the average age of pts being < 70 years. This is the first study to examine the effect of a purely pharmacist-led intervention.
Ekman, et al. Eur Heart J 1998 (Sweden)	**158** HF pts aged > 65 years and admitted to the medical wards of a	Nurse-monitored outpatient programme of care	Hospital readmissions over a mean follow-up	There were no differences between groups.	Although described as a feasibility study, this was a randomised study

(Continued)

Table 3.1 continued

Study	Study cohort	Study intervention	Major end points	Results	Comments
	university-affiliated hospital and discharged to home.	for symptom management plus telephone follow-up.	period of **5 months**.		where a large proportion of pts in the active group were not exposed to it. Overall, a poorly designed study.
Cline, et al. *Heart* 1998 (Sweden)	**190** HF pts aged 65–84 years admitted to a university-affiliated hospital and discharged to home.	In-hospital counselling, plus incremental follow-up at a nurse-led, heart failure-specific outpatient clinic.	Time to readmission, duration of hospital stay and healthcare costs within **1 year**.	Mean time to first admission was prolonged in study pts (P < 0·05). There were no significant differences in survival, hospital stay, and healthcare costs at 1 year – all favoured study pts.	Pts were not specifically selected on the basis of risk. However, there were strong trends in favour of study pts in all outcomes studied and Type II error was likely.
Stewart, et al. *Arch Intern Med* 1998 (Australia)	**97** HF pts admitted to a tertiary referral hospital in Adelaide, who participated in a larger study of a home intervention (n = 762).	A combination of pre-discharge education and a home visit by a nurse and pharmacist.	Event-free survival and hospital readmissions within **6 months**.	Pts in the study group had fewer primary events (37 vs. 68 events: P < 0·05) and fewer days of hospitalisation (261 vs. 452: P < 0·05).	This post-hoc analysis suggested that a non-specific multidisciplinary intervention was most effective in pts with HF.
Rich, et al. *N Engl J Med* 1995 (USA)	**282** "high risk" HF pts aged ≥ 70 years from the medical units of the Washington University Medical Center.	Nurse-led multi-disciplinary intervention involving both home and clinic visits.	Event-free survival, rate of readmission, quality of life, and cost of care within **3 months**.	Event-free survival favoured study pts (P = 0·09). Study pts had fewer readmissions, better quality of life and fewer healthcare costs (P < 0·05).	This was the first properly powered and randomised study of a nurse-led intervention in CHF. Although study follow-up was limited to 3 months, longer-term benefits were shown.

NS = non significant; NYHA = New York Heart Association; HF = heart failure; HR = hazard ratio

randomised studies with rigorous descriptions of their research methods and study follow-up. Their publication represented a contribution to the literature in addition to being distinct programmes of care that can be readily adapted and applied in different healthcare systems to typically older patients at high risk for subsequent morbidity and mortality.

In the first properly powered and conducted study of its type, Rich and colleagues[31] found that a nurse-led, multidisciplinary intervention (which involved a component of home visits) had beneficial effects as regards rates of hospital readmission, quality of life and cost of care within 90 days of discharge among "high risk" chronic heart failure patients. The intervention consisted of comprehensive education of the patient and family, a prescribed diet, social service consultation and planning for an early discharge, optimisation of pharmacotherapy, and intensive home and clinic-based follow-up with frequent telephone contact. At 90 days, survival without readmission was achieved in 91 of 142 (64%) intervention patients compared to 75 of 140 (54%) control patients ($P = 0.09$). There were 94 v 53 readmissions in the control and intervention groups respectively ($P = 0.02$). These readmissions equated to a total of 865 v 556 days of hospitalisation (a 36% reduction) or 6.2 v 3.9 days per patient ($P = 0.04$).[31]

Following post hoc analyses of a large-scale randomised controlled study of chronically ill patients with a mixture of cardiac and non-cardiac disease states,[67] which showed that a nurse-led, multidisciplinary, home-based intervention was most effective in heart failure,[49,53] Stewart and colleagues prospectively examined a more specific form of a nurse-led, home based intervention in 200 patients (100 in each group).[29] During six months follow-up the primary end point occurred more frequently in the usual care group (129 v 77 primary events; $P = 0.02$). More intervention patients remained event-free (38 v 51; $P = 0.04$). Overall, there were fewer unplanned readmissions (68 v 118; $P = 0.03$) and associated days of hospitalisation (460 v 1173; $P = 0.02$) among patients assigned to the study intervention.[29]

As described in Chapter 4, Lynda Blue and colleagues[28] studied a more intensive home based intervention than that applied in Australia, with 165 patients admitted to a tertiary referral hospital in Glasgow, Scotland. Compared with usual care, those patients exposed to the study intervention had fewer readmissions for any reason (86 v 114; $P = 0.02$), fewer admissions for heart failure (19 v 45; $P < 0.001$) and fewer days of hospitalisation (mean 3.4 v 7.5 days; $P = 0.005$).[28]

Recently, Riegel and colleagues[57] undertook the first appropriately powered randomised study of telephonic case management (i.e. no formalised clinic or home visits) of patients with heart failure. Although a significant proportion of patients were lost to follow-up, it still represents a particularly large study with outcome data reported on

242 patients. The effect of this intervention on heart failure related outcomes was significant with a 50% reduction in readmissions and associated stay. However, the overall effect on all-cause stay was non-significant, with a 30% reduction relative to usual care.[57] This latest study whilst confirming the general utility of phone follow-up (particularly in the absence of other forms of intervention) reinforces the benefits of a more flexible programme based on one to one contact with the patient to address problems not necessarily specific to heart failure.

Longer-term impact

Nearly all of the studies described above have been limited in follow-up and the potential for patients in the study arms of these studies to accumulate more outcomes in the longer term relative to usual care (thereby bridging the initial gap in healthcare utilisation rates and attenuating initial cost benefits) represents an important caveat in assessing their relative value. The ultimate aim of course is reduced healthcare costs over the typical lifespan of the target patient cohort. For example, with the exception of the 10-year follow-up of the original Cooperative North Scandinavian Enalapril Survival Study (CONSENSUS) cohort,[68] there are very few studies to suggest that clinically effective treatments in heart failure (including β-blockers and spironolactone) are associated with sustained cost benefits – particularly when such treatments are associated with prolonged survival and therefore the opportunity for further morbidity still exists. With this major caveat in mind, we recently examined the longer-term effects of the nurse-led, multidisciplinary, home-based intervention on the 298 Australian patients participating in the two randomised studies outlined in Table 3.1.[29,49] Median study follow-up was for 4·2 years and ranged from 3 to 6 years post-discharge.[60] During prolonged follow-up, nearly all patients were either hospitalised or died. A total of 96 of 148 patients (65%) in the usual care group died. In comparison a total of 83 of 149 patients (56%) subject to the study intervention had died and this was independently associated with a 28% relative risk reduction in mortality (P < 0·05). Despite the more prolonged survival in the study group (equivalent to an additional 817 months of survival overall) initially observed benefits in respect to recurrent hospital stay persisted over the longer term. Moreover, although the relative difference in recurrent stay fell from 60% at six months to 22% at three years, an absolute cost difference was preserved with healthcare costs remaining substantially lower in the longer term (see Figure 3.2).[60]

New directions

In recent years there has been increasing interest in applying interactive home telemonitoring to enhance surveillance for clinical

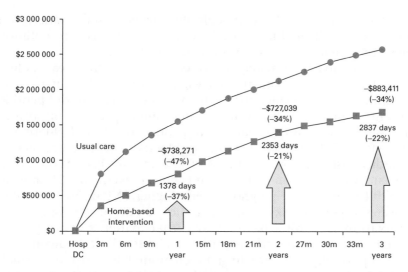

Figure 3.2 Economic impact of a nurse-led heart failure programme via a reduction in recurrent hospital stay over three years[60]

deterioration/sub-optimal control of chronic heart failure. With the availability of more cost-effective and user-friendly equipment (costs still remain prohibitive and the information technology revolution has yet to reach its promised potential) the potential for applying technology that allows telephonic transmission of key data (for example vital signs, weight, and ECG) from the patient's home to the physician/nurse has increased. Following on from a positive pilot study reported by Shah and colleagues,[69] the recently reported Trans European Network Homecare Monitoring Study (TEN-HMS)[70] randomised 427 patients to three study arms – usual care, usual care supplemented by regular telephonic contact with a specialist nurse, or telemonitoring. After 400 days follow-up, the reported mortality rate was 26% in the usual care group compared to 15% in those supported via telephone and 13% in those exposed to telemonitoring (P < 0·03 for both comparisons). The total number of readmissions in the telemonitoring group was greater than in the nurse-led telephonic support group but total numbers of days in hospital were slightly less. A full analysis of this study pending publication of a full study report will obviously need to be made. However, telemonitoring clearly has a potential role in the proactive management of heart failure and similar trials are beginning to appear in the literature.[71] There is little doubt that many will view interactive monitoring as a means to replace existing forms of follow-up. However, apart from obvious issues relating to cost and the preparedness and ability of older patients to tolerate computerised surveillance, it is more than likely that a combination of technologically advanced surveillance, and nursing care delivered by specialist nurses, will be used to optimise the management of chronic heart failure in the future.

A new approach to managing patients with chronic heart failure advocated by Troughton and colleagues from Christchurch, New Zealand, based on measurement of blood natriuretic peptide concentrations, may have a more immediate impact on this area of clinical practice.[72] B-type natriuretic peptide (BNP) and N-terminal pro-BNP (NT-BNP) are secreted into the blood by the heart as a marker of cardiac distress. Concentrations of BNP and NT-BNP in the blood correlate with the haemodynamic and clinical severity of CHF and are powerful predictors of prognosis, i.e. a higher BNP or NT-BNP value indicates a greater risk of hospitalisation or death.[73–77] Two recent observational studies have shown that patients with greater reductions in BNP after treatment have a better clinical outcome.[78,79] More importantly still, the Christchurch group has carried out a small randomised study to test the hypothesis that treatment adjusted to lower NT-BNP might lead to a better outcome than medical therapy prescribed in the usual way.[72] This pilot study enrolled 69 patients. Lower blood NT-BNP concentrations were attained in the guided therapy group and these patients had a lower risk of the primary composite end point of worsening CHF, hospital readmissions, or cardiovascular death.[72] After a mean follow-up of 9·6 months, there were 19 events in the NT-BNP compared to 54 in the usual care group (P = 0·02). There were 1 and 7 deaths, 11 and 26 out-patient heart failure events and 5 and 13 CHF hospitalisations in the guided therapy and usual care groups, respectively. Currently, these pilot data are being further investigated in appropriately powered randomised studies.

Meta-analyses

A recently published meta-analysis of disease management programmes in heart failure (not necessarily involving specialist nurse management) demonstrated that such programmes are associated with an overall reduced risk of hospitalisation (RR = 0·87, 95% CI 0·79–0·96).[80] A more contemporary and specific meta-analysis of 19 randomised controlled trials involving approximately 1900 patients presented at the 2003 European Society of Cardiology meeting demonstrated that post-discharge heart failure programmes predominantly involving specialist heart failure nurses are associated with a 30% reduced risk of hospital readmission (odds ratio 0·70, 95% CI 0·58–0·85: P < 0·001), a 34% reduced risk of death or hospital readmission (odds ratio 0·66, 95% CI 0·54 – 0·81: P < 0·001) and, most remarkably, a 20% reduced risk of all-cause mortality (odds ratio 0·80, 95% CI 0·65 – 0·99: P < 0·05).[81] Remarkably, this analysis demonstrated that such programmes prevent a total of 160 events (comprising deaths and heart failure related hospitalisations) per 1000 patient years of treatment as compared to a range of 28–63 events prevented by ACE inhibitors, β-blockers, or digoxin.[81]

Based on these key studies, a further careful interpretation of the literature to date, and these meta-analyses, it would appear that these programmes, particularly those that involve a component of home-based intervention and nurse-led coordination of multidisciplinary care, have the potential to achieve five important goals in the management of heart failure:

1. prolonged event-free (hospitalisation or death) survival
2. reduced readmission rates
3. reduced multiple readmissions – i.e. a "peak" effect on the high cost/high utilisation patients
4. improved quality of life
5. reduced overall costs – mainly due to a reduction in recurrent length of stay in lower cost units (for example fewer days in intensive/coronary care units).

These represent substantial benefits on both an individual and a population based level. From an economic perspective, however, the most important indicator is the effect of these programmes on recurrent hospital stay (the most expensive component of heart failure related health care[82]). Figure 3.3 presents a summary of this type of data from a range of studies expressed as days of readmission/ patient. A number of these studies recruited "low risk patients" (for example younger patients). However, the expected trend of "accumulative" hospital use over time (i.e. depending on the duration of follow-up) is evident. As expected, the studies associated with the greatest effect on recurrent stay were those involving a component of home-based intervention (USA A and D, England, Scotland, and Australia A and B).

Conclusions

Considering the enormity of the epidemic of heart failure and the cost burden it imposes on nearly all developed countries, there is clearly a need to create and apply new models of health care that will provide benefits on both an individual and a population based level. While the application of proven pharmacological agents should be incorporated into the gold standard care of patients with heart failure they form only part of the solution. In recent years, there has been increasing evidence to suggest that programmes involving specialist nurse management can improve health outcomes in typically old and

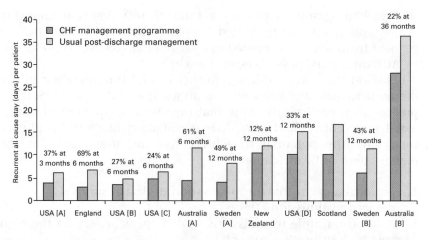

Figure 3.3 Direct comparison of recurrent all-cause hospital stay in a range of randomised trials of post-discharge programmes for chronic heart failure management according to length of follow up

fragile patients with heart failure. As described in more detail in Chapter 5, based on clinically significant reductions in recurrent hospital stay (the predominant component of heart failure related expenditure) these programmes are likely to be remarkably cost-effective when applied on a formal basis. Clearly there is scope for more research in this area. However, the data remain compelling both on an individual and on a population basis. As such, neither our patients nor our healthcare systems can do without nurse-led programmes of post-discharge care to optimise the management of heart failure while providing individualised care and attention and improving subsequent health outcomes.

References

1   Petrie MC, Dawson NF, Murdoch DR, Davie AP, McMurray JJ. Failure of women's hearts. *Circulation* 1999;**99**:2334–41.
2   Petrie MC, Berry C, Stewart S, McMurray JJ. Failing ageing hearts. *Eur Heart J* 2001;**22**:1978–90.
3   Stewart S, Hart C, Hole DJ, McMurray JJ. The incidence and natural history of heart failure during 20-year follow-up of the 15 406 men and women: the Renfrew/Paisley Study. *Circulation* 2001;**104**:II-826.
4   McKee PA, Castelli WP, McNamara PM, Kannel WB. The natural history of congestive heart failure: the Framingham study. *N Engl J Med* 1971;**285**:1441–6.
5   McMurray JJ, Stewart S. Epidemiology, aetiology and prognosis of heart failure. *Heart* 2000;**83**:596–602.
6   MacDowall P, Kalra PA, O'Donoghue DJ, Waldek S, Mamtora H, Brown K. Risk of morbidity from renovascular disease in elderly patients with congestive cardiac failure. *Lancet* 1998;**352**:13–16.
7   Mitka M. Researchers probe anemia–heart failure link. *JAMA* 2003;**290**:1834–5.

8 Clarke KW, Gray D, Hampton JR. Evidence of inadequate investigation and treatment of patients with heart failure. *Br Heart J* 1994;**71**:584–7.

9 Juenger J, Schellberg D, Kraemer S, et al. Health related quality of life in patients with congestive heart failure: comparison with other chronic diseases and relation to functional variables. *Heart* 2002;**87**:235–41.

10 Stewart S, Demers C, Murdoch DR, et al. Substantial between-hospital variation in outcome following first emergency admission with heart failure. *Eur Heart J* 2002;**23**: 650–7.

11 Boulay F, Berthier F, Sisteron O, et al. Seasonal variation in chronic heart failure hospitalizations and mortality in France. *Circulation* 1999;**100**:280–6.

12 Stewart S, MacIntyre K, Capewell S, McMurray JJ. Heart failure in a cold climate: seasonal variation in heart failure-related morbidity and mortality. *J Am Coll Cardiol* 2002;**39**:760–6.

13 Stewart S, MacIntyre K, Hole DJ, et al. More 'malignant' than cancer? Five-year survival following a first admission for heart failure. *Eur J Heart Fail* 2001;**3**:315–22.

14 Cowie MR, Wood DA, Coats AJS, et al. Survival of patients with a new diagnosis of heart failure: a population based study. *Heart* 2001;**83**:505–10·

15 MacIntyre K, Capewell S, Stewart S, et al. Evidence of improving prognosis in heart failure: trends in case fatality in 66 547 patients hospitalized between 1986 and 1995. *Circulation* 2000;**102**:1126–31.

16 Luttik M, Jaarsma T, Van Veldhuisen DJ. Quality of life of caregivers is worse compared to patients with congestive heart failure. *Eur Heart J* 2003;**24**:64.

17 Wolinski FD, Smith DM, Stump TE, Everhoge JM, Lubitz RM. The sequelae of hospitalisation for congestive heart failure among older adults. *J Am Geriatr Soc* 1997;**45**:558–63.

18 Krumholz HM, Parent EM, Tu N, et al. Readmission after hospitalization for congestive heart failure among Medicare beneficiaries. *Arch Intern Med* 1997;**157**: 99–104.

19 Vinson JM, Rich MW, Sperry JC, Shah AS, McNamara T. Early readmission of elderly patients with congestive heart failure. *J Am Geriatr Soc* 1990;**38**:1290–5.

20 Happ MB, Naylor MD, Roe-Prior P. Factors contributing to rehospitalization of elderly patients with heart failure. *J Cardiovasc Nurs* 1997;**11**:75–84.

21 Michalsen A, Konig G, Thimme W. Preventable causative factors leading to hospital admission with decompensated heart failure. *Heart* 1998;**80**:437–41.

22 Stewart S, Horowitz JD. Detecting early clinical deterioration in chronic heart failure patients post-acute hospitalisation – a critical component of multidisciplinary, home-based intervention? *Eur J Heart Fail* 2002;**4**:345–51.

23 Moser K, Mann DL. Improving outcomes in heart failure: it's not unusual beyond usual care. *Circulation* 2002;**105**:2810–12.

24 Tunstall-Pedoe H, Kuulasmaa K, Mahonen M, et al. Contribution of trends in survival and coronary-event rates to changes in coronary heart disease mortality: 10-year results from 37 WHO MONICA project populations. *Lancet* 1999;**353**: 1547–57.

25 Capewell S, Beaglehole R, Seddon M, McMurray JJ. Explanation for the decline in coronary heart disease mortality rates in Auckland, New Zealand, between 1982 and 1993. *Circulation* 2000;**102**:1511–6.

26 McMurray JJ, Stewart S. Nurse led, multidisciplinary intervention in chronic heart failure. *Heart* 1998;**80**:430–1.

27 Rich MW. Heart failure disease management: a critical review. *J Card Fail* 1999;**5**: 64–75.

28 Yusuf S, Sleight P, Pogue J, et al. Effects of an angiotensin-converting-enzyme inhibitor, ramipril, on cardiovascular events in high-risk patients. The Heart Outcomes Prevention Evaluation Study Investigators. *N Engl J Med* 2001;**342**: 145–53.

29 Stewart S, Marley JE, Horowitz JD. Effects of a multidisciplinary, home-based intervention on unplanned readmissions and survival among patients with chronic congestive heart failure: a randomised controlled study. *Lancet* 1999;**354**:1077–83.

30 Blue L, Lang E, McMurray JJ, et al. Randomised controlled trial of specialist nurse intervention in heart failure. *BMJ* 2001;**323**:715–18.

31 Rich MW, Beckham V, Wittenberg C, Leven CL, Freedland KE, Carney RM. A multidisciplinary intervention to prevent the readmission of elderly patients with congestive heart failure. *N Engl J Med* 1995;**333**:1190–5.

32 Mark DB. Economics of treating heart failure. *Am J Cardiol* 1997;**80**:33H–38H.
33 Wright SP, Walsh H, Ingley SA, *et al.* Uptake of self-management strategies in a heart failure management programme. *Eur J Heart Fail* 2003;**5**:371–80.
34 Gattis WA, Hasselblad V, Whellan DJ, O'Connor CM. Reduction in heart failure events by the addition of a clinical pharmacist to the heart failure management team: Results of the Pharmacist in Heart Failure Assessment Recommendation and Monitoring (PHARM) Study. *Arch Intern Med* 1999;**159**:1939–45.
35 Kornowski R, Zeeli D, Averbuch M, *et al.* Intensive home-care surveillance prevents hospitalization and improves morbidity rates among elderly patients with severe congestive heart failure. *Am Heart J* 1995;**129**:762–6.
36 West JA, Miller NH, Parker KM, *et al.* A comprehensive management system for heart failure improves clinical outcomes and reduces medical resource utilization. *Am J Cardiol* 1997;**79**:58–63.
37 Fonarow GC, Stevenson LW, Walden JA, *et al.* Impact of a comprehensive heart failure management program on hospital readmission and functional status of patients with advanced heart failure. *J Am Coll Cardiol* 1997;**30**:725–32.
38 Shah NB, Der E, Ruggerio C, Heindenreich PA, Massie BM. Prevention of hospitalizations for heart failure with an interactive home monitoring program. *Am Heart J* 1998;**135**:373–8.
39 Jerant AF, Azari R, Nesbitt TS. Reducing the cost of frequent hospital admissions for congestive heart failure: a randomized trial of a home telecare intervention. *Med Care* 2001;**39**:1234–45.
40 Cordisco ME, Benjaminovitz A, Hammond K, Mancini D. Use of telemonitoring to decrease the rate of hospitalization in patients with severe congestive heart failure. *Am J Cardiol* 1999;**84**:860–2.
41 Roglieri J, Futterman R, McDonough KL, *et al.* Disease management interventions to improve outcomes in congestive heart failure. *Am J Manag Care* 1997;**3**:1831–9.
42 Cintron G, Bigas C, Linares E, Aranda JM, Hernandez E. Nurse practitioner role in a chronic congestive heart failure clinic: in-hospital time, costs and patient satisfaction. *Heart Lung* 1993;**12**:237–40.
43 Lasater M. The effect of a nurse-managed CHF clinic on patient readmission and length of stay. *Home Healthc Nurse* 1996;**14**:351–6.
44 Hanumanthu S, Butler J, Chomsky D, David S, Wilson JR. Effect of a heart failure program on hospitalization frequency and exercise tolerance. *Circulation* 1997;**96**: 2842–8.
45 Dahl J, Penque S. The effects of an advanced practice nurse-directed heart failure program. *Nurse Pract* 2000;**25**:61–77.
46 Holst DP, Kaye D, Richardson M, *et al.* Improved outcomes from a comprehensive management system for heart failure. *Eur J Heart Fail* 2001;**3**:619–25.
47 Macko MJ. Evaluation of cost and hospitalisation outcomes from a community case management programme serving heart failure clients. *J Card Fail* 1998;**4**:59.
48 McDonald K, Ledwidge M, Cahill J, *et al.* Elimination of early rehospitalization in a randomized, controlled trial of multidisciplinary care in a high-risk, elderly heart failure population: the potential contributions of specialist care, clinical stability and optimal angiotensin-converting enzyme inhibitor dose at discharge. *Eur J Heart Fail* 2001;**3**:209–15.
49 Stewart S, Pearson S, Horowitz JD. Effects of a home-based intervention among patients with congestive heart failure discharged from acute hospital care. *Arch Intern Med* 1998;**158**:1067–72.
50 Cline CM, Israelsson BY, Willenheimer RB, *et al.* Cost effective management programme for heart failure reduces hospitalisation. *Heart* 1998;**80**:442–6.
51 Ekman I, Andersson B, Ehnfors M, *et al.* Feasibility of a nurse-monitored, outpatient-care programme for elderly patients with moderate-to-severe, chronic heart failure. *Eur Heart J* 1998;**19**:1254–60.
52 Oddone EZ, Weinberger M, Giobbie-Hurder A, Landsman P, Henderson W. Enhanced access to primary care for patients with congestive heart failure. Veterans Affairs Cooperative Study Group on Primary Care and Hospital Readmission. *Eff Clin Pract* 1999;**2**:201–9.
53 Stewart S, Vandenbroek A, Pearson S, Horowitz J. Prolonged beneficial effects of a home-based intervention on unplanned readmissions and mortality among patients with congestive heart failure. *Arch Intern Med* 1999;**159**:257–61.

54 Jaarsma T, Halfens R, Huijer Abu-Saad H, *et al.* Effects of education and support on self-care and resource utilization in patients with heart failure. *Eur Heart J* 1999; 20:673–82.

55 Doughty RN, Wright SP, Walsh HJ, *et al.* Randomized, controlled trial of integrated heart failure management: The Auckland Heart Failure Management Study. *Eur Heart J* 2002;23:139–46.

56 Krumholz HM, Amatruda J, Smith GL, *et al.* Randomized trial of an education and support intervention to prevent readmission of patients with heart failure. *J Am Coll Cardiol* 2002;39:83–9.

57 Riegel B, Carlson B, Kopp Z, *et al.* Effect of a standardized nurse case-management telephone intervention on resource use in patients with chronic heart failure. *Arch Intern Med* 2002;162:705–12.

58 Harrison MB, Browne GB, Roberts J, Tugwell P, Gafni A, Graham ID. Quality of life of individuals with heart failure: a randomized trial of the effectiveness of two models of hospital-to-home transition. *Med Care* 2002;40:271–82.

59 Kasper EK, Gerstenblith G, Hefter G, *et al.* A randomized trial of the efficacy of multidisciplinary care in heart failure outpatients at high risk of hospital readmission. *J Am Coll Cardiol* 2002;39:471–80.

60 Stewart S, Horowitz JD. Home-based intervention in congestive heart failure: long-term implications on readmission and survival. *Circulation* 2002;105:2861–6.

61 Strömberg A, Martensson J, Fridlund B, Levin LA, Karlsson JE, Dahlstrom U. Nurse-led heart failure clinics improve survival and self-care behaviour in patients with heart failure: results from a prospective randomised trial. *Eur Heart J* 2003; 24:1014–23.

62 Naylor M, Brooten D, Jones R, Lavizzo-Mourey R, Mezey M, Pauly M. Comprehensive discharge planning for the hospitalized elderly. A randomized clinical trial. *Ann Intern Med* 1994;120:999–1006.

63 Naylor MD, Brooten D, Cambell R, *et al.* Comprehensive discharge planning and home follow-up of hospitalized elders: a randomized clinical trial. *JAMA* 1999; 281:613–20.

64 Fitzgerald JF, Smith DM, Martin DK, Freedman JA, Katz BP. A case manager intervention to reduce readmissions. *Arch Intern Med* 1994;154:1721–9.

65 Moser DK, Macko MJ, Worster P. Community case management decreases rehospitalisation rates and costs, and improves quality of life in heart failure patients with preserved and non-preserved left ventricular function: A randomized controlled trial. *Circulation* 2000;102:II–749.

66 Thompson DR, Roebuck A, Stewart S. Effects of a nurse-led, clinic and home-based intervention on recurrent hospital use in chronic heart failure. *Eur Heart J* 2003; 24:485.

67 Stewart S, Pearson S, Luke CG, Horowitz JD. Effects of home-based intervention on unplanned readmissions and out-of-hospital deaths. *J Am Geriatr Soc* 1998;46: 174–80.

68 Swedberg K, Kjekshus J, Snapinn S. Long-term survival in severe heart failure in patients with enalapril. Ten year follow-up of CONSENSUS I. *Eur Heart J* 1999;20:136–9.

69 Shah NB, Der E, Ruggerio C, Heidenreich PA, Massie BM. Prevention of hospitalizations for heart failure with an interactive home monitoring program. *Am Heart J* 1998;135:373–8.

70 Coletta AP, Louis AA, Clark AL, *et al.* Clinical trials update from the European Society of Cardiology: CARMEN, EARTH, OPTIMAAL, ACE, TEN-HMS, MAGIC, SOLVD-X and PATH-CHF II. *Eur J Heart Fail* 2002;4:661–6.

71 Williams RE, Acker K, Cashy J. Prospective, randomized, controlled trial (RCT) of an automated daily heart failure telemonitoring program. *J Card Fail* 2003; 9:S63.

72 Troughton RW, Frampton CM, Yandle TG, *et al.* Treatment of heart failure guided by plasma aminoterminal brain natriuretic peptide (N-BNP) concentrations. *Lancet* 2000;355:1126–30.

73 Berger R, Stanek B, Frey B, *et al.* B-type natriuretic peptides (BNP and PRO-BNP) predict longterm survival in patients with advanced heart failure treated with atenolol. *J Heart Lung Transplant* 2001;20:251.

74 McDonagh TA, Cunningham AD, Morrison CE, *et al.* Left ventricular dysfunction, natriuretic peptides, and mortality in an urban population. *Heart* 2001;86:21–6.

75 Berger R, Huelsman M, Strecker K, *et al*. B-type natriuretic peptide predicts sudden death in patients with chronic heart failure. *Circulation* 2002;**105**:2392–7.

76 Anand IS, Fisher LD, Chiang YT, *et al*. Changes in brain natriuretic peptide and norepinephrine over time and mortality and morbidity in the Valsartan Heart Failure Trial (Val-HeFT). *Circulation* 2003;**107**:1278–83.

77 Fisher C, Berry C, Blue L, Morton JJ, McMuray JJ. N-terminal pro B type natriuretic peptide, but not the new putative cardiac hormone relaxin, predicts prognosis in patients with chronic heart failure. *Heart* 2003;**89**:879–81.

78 Cheng V, Kazanagra R, Garcia A, *et al*. A rapid bedside test for B-type peptide predicts treatment outcomes in patients admitted for decompensated heart failure: a pilot study. *J Am Coll Cardiol* 2001;**37**:386–91.

79 Bettencourt P, Ferreira S, Azevedo A, Ferreira A. Preliminary data on the potential usefulness of B type natriuretic peptide levels in predicting outcome after hospital discharge in patients with heart failure. *Am J Med* 2002;**113**:215–9.

80 McAlister FA, Lawson FM, Teo KK, Armstrong PW. A systematic review of randomized trials of disease management programs in heart failure. *Am J Med* 2001;**110**:378–84.

81 Stewart S, Berry C, McMurray JJ. Multidisciplinary intervention in congestive heart failure – does it reduce morbidity and mortality? *Eur Heart J* 2003;**24**:65.

82 Stewart S, Jenkins A, Buchan S, McGuire A, Capewell S, McMurray JJ. The current cost of heart failure to the National Health Service in the UK. *Eur J Heart Fail* 2002;**4**: 361–71.

Section 2:
The Glasgow experience

4: Glasgow Heart Failure Liaison Service: a model for future services

LYNDA BLUE

Introduction

As described in Chapter 3, many patients with chronic heart failure have limited knowledge of both their condition and its treatment, and are frequently non-compliant or self-adjust increasingly more complex medication regimens.[1] Combined with inherent inefficiencies in most healthcare systems incapable of managing patients with complex chronic disease states or ensuring that appropriate treatment is prescribed, as described in Chapter 1, morbidity and mortality rates remain unacceptably high. The UK healthcare system, as in other developed countries, is generally inflexible with a lack of resources (both in respect to time and money) to meet the exacting needs of patients and families affected by chronic heart failure and the complex issues it engenders. Although some admissions associated with chronic heart failure are appropriate and desirable for optimal management, there has been increasing evidence to support the notion that a substantial proportion of hospitalisations in typically old and fragile patients are preventable.[2,3] In Glasgow, Scotland it was recognised that heart failure nurse specialists had the potential to alleviate the overall burden of heart failure by limiting costly admissions, in addition to improving quality of life on an individual basis by providing more tailored and attentive care. Key studies described in Chapter 3 showed that home based, specialist nurse-led, multidisciplinary intervention can significantly improve health outcomes in patients with severe chronic heart failure.[4-6] The studies also provided evidence, in addition to our own efforts, to develop an effective city-wide service that would bridge the divide between research and practice and meet the particular needs of patients with this syndrome living in the city of Glasgow.

From research to practice

The Glasgow Heart Failure Liaison Service was formally established following a positive randomised controlled trial undertaken during 1997–99 and described in more detail in Chapter 3.[6] Briefly, the aim of the trial was to determine whether home based nurse intervention, in addition to conventional care, could reduce unnecessary hospital readmission and improve quality of life for patients with chronic heart failure secondary to left ventricular systolic dysfunction after hospital discharge. The trial showed a significant reduction in readmissions and hospital bed days related to heart failure. As a result of the positive outcome from the trial and evidence from supporting literature the Health Authority in Glasgow provided funding for a nurse-led, city-wide Heart Failure Liaison Service based on the study model.

It is worth noting that the decision to translate research into practice, with the provision of sufficient funds and time to develop sustainable resources, remains the exception to the rule even in an environment of more compelling evidence – particularly in relation to cost-effectiveness.

Service description

The Glasgow Heart Failure Liaison Service formally commenced operation in July 2000. A staged approach, with planned incremental introduction of the service across five key sites in the city over a period of 13 months, ensured sufficient time to develop, test, and adjust service protocols. Currently, there are 7·5 whole-time equivalent (WTE) heart failure specialist nurses employed by the local primary care organisation. All are based in the five adult acute hospital sites (1·5 WTE per site) serving the local population of around one million people.

In developing the Glasgow service we adopted the same inclusion criteria as used in the randomised controlled trial – patients with chronic heart failure secondary to left ventricular systolic dysfunction determined by echocardiography, radionuclide ventriculography, or angiography. The exclusion criteria include:

- patients unwilling to have this support (an isolated few)
- other immediately life threatening illness, for example advanced malignancy
- acute myocardial infarction unless the patient has previously had the support of the service
- living outside the Greater Glasgow Health Authority area
- discharge to long-term care

- patients with a history of abusive behaviour towards health care professionals.

When establishing a service it is important to fine-tune already established procedures and protocols. It is also extremely important to take into account the learning needs and skills of newly appointed specialist nurses. This led to our decision, for example, to concentrate initially on only those patients with chronic heart failure secondary to left ventricular systolic dysfunction as opposed to those patients with preserved systolic function/diastolic dysfunction or primary valvular dysfunction.

Key considerations in establishing a heart failure service

Creating a new health care service is a complex and time-consuming process. It should come as no surprise, therefore, that once the decision was made to create the Glasgow service there were many difficulties and obstacles to overcome. Careful planning and consideration of the purpose and scope of the service was required as was a change in mind-set from researching a potentially useful intervention to one that could be replicated and sustained in a cost-effective manner throughout the city.

The box below outlines the key considerations that underpinned the establishment of this successful service. As can be appreciated, there were many things to consider but good planning is always time well spent. Some of the most important points considered included the limitations of the pre-existing healthcare system and the most practical means by which health outcomes can be improved. The following sections describe the key components of the Glasgow Heart Failure Liaison Service. It was implemented to overcome the limitations of the healthcare system and improve the unacceptably high morbidity and mortality rates usually associated with chronic heart failure.

Key considerations in establishing a heart failure service

Formulating a strategy

- Devise a strategy to present to the relevant Health Authority (this is easier to achieve if there is a good evidence base). The strategy should underpin local implementation of any national guidelines; for example, in the United Kingdom we used the National Service Framework and Scottish Intercollegiate Guidelines Network

- Interest a few enthusiasts and influential leaders
- Identify stakeholders and form a steering group with representation from all stakeholder groups, healthcare professionals, and managers from hospital and community (ensure all stakeholders are involved)
- If possible try a pilot first to show the service can work, and its benefits can help secure further resources
- Plan for recurrent resources from the start
- Ensure model of care suits local environment

Defining the strategy

- Decide priorities and agree purpose of the service
- Develop precise and realistic aims and objectives
- Draw up clear protocols and guidelines which have been agreed by all the key stakeholders and reflect local and national guidelines
- Define referral criteria – which patients, and how will they be referred?
- Develop mechanisms to identify eligible patients and how they will be referred to the service
- Ensure support from key players, for example general practitioner/primary care physician, hospital physician, including a system in place to access specialist advice for unstable patients
- Assess possible numbers of patients
- Identify numbers of specialist nurses required and what grades
- Identify other support required, for example administration, management, financial

Planning the practical issues

- Incremental approach valuable (sort out teething problems when they occur)
- Establish formal links with other relevant healthcare services
- Clarify role with other healthcare professionals to avoid inappropriate referrals
- Ensure cooperation from all hospital physicians (not just the enthusiasts)
- Know limitation of numbers to avoid overloading the system
- Develop a patient information book
- Regular evaluation and audit (see Chapter 6)
- Regular review of service protocols and guidelines
- Patient/carer satisfaction (see Chapter 8)
- Review resources
- Ensure practice keeps pace with research
- Set realistic goals on future development
- Budgeting and resources (see box below)

Budgeting and resources

- Cost for salary and overheads of specialist nurses (built in cover for sickness, annual leave, study leave, etc)
- Office and/or clinic space and equipment
- Transport (for example supplying a car with ongoing travel costs)
- Communication (for example phone, mobile phone, fax, paperwork, computing)

- Equipment (for example weighing scales for patients, venepuncture equipment, computer equipment)
- Additional investigations (for example laboratory costs)
- Referral costs to other professionals (for example dietician, pharmacist, social worker, audit personnel, information technology support)
- Patient information books
- Training costs (for example an induction programme, ongoing training and development)

Key elements of the Glasgow Heart Failure Liaison Service

The box below outlines the aims and philosophy of the Glasgow service. These cannot be met without implementation of the key elements that characterise this service.

Aims and philosophy of the Glasgow Heart Failure Liaison Service

Aims of the service

- To provide effective management for patients by working seamlessly across both the primary and secondary care sectors
- To reduce the level of unnecessary hospital readmissions
- To initiate appropriate pharmacological regimens
- To improve the quality of life for patients with chronic heart failure, as well as assessing and planning future care
- To impart information, advice, and support for both patients and carers

Patient-specific objectives

- To assess patients in their home environment and plan for their future needs in accordance with the service guidelines
- To review the prescribed medication regimen to ensure that patients receive appropriate pharmacotherapy in effective doses
- To work to agreed prescription guidelines drawn up in conjunction with general practitioners and cardiologists
- To monitor the patient's clinical status and blood chemistry following medication changes
- To ensure appropriate and effective communication between the patient, general practitioner, carer, ambulance services, hospital, social services, and all other health-care professionals involved in the patient's care
- To provide patients, families, and carers with tailored education, advice, and support
- To act as a resource for other healthcare professionals involved with the patient
- To advise the patient on lifestyle changes that would be advantageous to their health
- To encourage patients (and their family or carers as appropriate) to be actively involved in managing and monitoring their own care

- To provide easy access for patients, family, and carers to contact the specialist nurse in order to detect and treat early clinical deterioration before symptoms become severe

Service-specific objectives

- To ensure that the overall nursing and medical care provided keeps pace with research evidence (for example effect of telemonitoring systems and palliative care needs)
- To monitor, evaluate, and audit the service at regular intervals to ensure both a high standard of care and the effectiveness of the service as a whole in improving health outcomes.
- To facilitate effective links with other healthcare services relevant to the care of the patient with chronic heart failure (including palliative care services)

Protocols and guidelines

The specialist nurses who form the core of the service are specially trained in heart failure management (see Appendix 1) and work in conjunction with local general practitioners (primary care physicians) and cardiologists to optimise the management of patients with chronic heart failure after hospital discharge. Staff within the service work to agreed protocols and guidelines and have access to a cardiologist for specialist advice for patients experiencing problems or difficulties that are not documented in the medical therapy guidelines. There are slight variations in how the service operates at the five sites.

Not surprisingly, it is important to create clear guidelines for the pharmacological and non-pharmacological management of patients exposed to the service. The former is especially important if the specialist nurse is empowered to initiate and adjust pharmacotherapy. However, even if they are not, he or she should be in a position to evaluate the effectiveness of prescribed therapy and initiate changes (either directly or indirectly) if required. The dynamic and fluctuating nature of this syndrome means that the pharmacological agents described in Chapter 2 need to be continually evaluated and adjusted (refer to Chapter 9 for detailed information in this regard).

To enable specialist heart failure nurses to operate as autonomous practitioners there must be support from key players (for example general practitioner, hospital physician, and/or a cardiologist) and a system in place to access specialist advice for unstable patients. It is also valuable to have access to a multidisciplinary team (for example clinical psychologist, pharmacist, dietician, social services, physiotherapist, and palliative care teams, etc). At present this is a luxury for most healthcare professionals working in the heart failure world.

As a result of modern therapies the natural history of chronic heart failure can be altered for the better, but it can be extremely labour intensive and complex to initiate and manage patients on appropriate heart failure therapy. Many responsible physicians lack either time or knowledge to facilitate appropriate management of heart failure. A large component of the heart failure specialist nurse role is therefore to initiate, titrate, and monitor pharmacological therapy to ensure that patients receive therapy that is consistent with agreed medical therapy guidelines.

Identifying patients

At present patients in the Glasgow service are predominantly identified during a hospital admission with acute decompensated heart failure secondary to left ventricular systolic dysfunction. Unstable patients with a confirmed diagnosis of chronic heart failure attending physician-led outpatient clinics can also be referred. The majority of the patients are high risk, elderly patients with significant other co-morbidities and are a patient group who are generally under-represented in heart failure clinical trials. It is vital to ensure that other healthcare professionals and patients understand the role of the specialist heart failure nurse to avoid both inappropriate referrals and unrealistic expectations from healthcare professionals.

Patient follow-up

One of the greatest areas of uncertainty concerning this type of intervention is the exact level of follow-up. The level of follow-up can have a large effect on the size of the service and has proved problematic in Glasgow since acquiring additional funding has proved difficult. Within existing resources the question of whether the emphasis should be on fewer patients with extensive follow-up or more patients with a less extensive follow-up has still to be answered. Probably the best approach is to provide a "safety net" or core programme of intervention for patients enrolled into the service. For example, all patients recruited to the Glasgow service receive a minimum of two home visits within the first month following hospital discharge, the first visit being within one week of discharge. However, many patients require substantially more contact – especially in the initial post-discharge period (more details are provided in Chapter 6). Subsequent contacts are determined by individual patients' needs. Patients, carers, and other healthcare professionals can easily access the nurses in the service by telephone and all patients have a follow-up telephone call at three months.

Current research has shown that telephone contact with this group of patients can be effective in continuing the impact on reduction of hospitalisations and resource use.[7] Written communication detailing the intervention is distributed to relevant healthcare professionals and sent to the patient's hospital case notes (see Chapter 6).

Although a major aim of the service is to reduce hospitalisation rates, much emphasis is also placed on making a positive impact on the patients' quality of life and satisfaction with their healthcare.

Patient education and support

Many patients feel anxious and are unwell when they are in the hospital setting. From an educational point of view, therefore, it is an inopportune time to pass on vital information and expect it to be remembered and/or valued. It is usually only when patients return home that they are able to formulate questions about their condition and seek to clarify treatment options. Following hospital discharge it is therefore beneficial for patients to be seen as soon as possible by the heart failure nurse specialist who can provide information, advice and support as well as assessing and planning future care.

Erhardt and colleagues have demonstrated that patients with heart failure need continuous, long-term support outside the hospital environment. It is therefore essential that a system is designed to provide patients with optimal care after discharge.[8] In providing repeat home visits and telephone follow-up (both nurse and patient initiated) the Glasgow service provides such long-term support.

Patient information book

Patients (especially the elderly) have difficulty in remembering the details of their condition and their treatment, especially when their pharmacological regimen is adjusted on a continuous basis in response to their heart failure status. Healthcare professionals also have difficulty in tracking the progress of the heart failure patient and appreciate a concise but accurate summary of both the patient and their treatment. A good way of facilitating both the patient's understanding of their condition and treatment and the healthcare professional's management of the heart failure is to provide the patient with an information book. This should both be educational and represent a record of their progress and treatment. Patients in the Glasgow service are provided with a patient information book prior to hospital discharge. This book has proved to be extremely valuable in providing detailed information about heart failure and its treatment, backing up verbal information the patient has initially received, and giving clear information for patients and carers on when and from whom to seek advice.

It is vital patients and their carers are provided with clear advice about what to do, and whom to contact, if their condition deteriorates. A study by Michalsen and colleagues showed that, despite progressive symptoms, patients often do not obtain prompt and adequate intervention. Nearly 80% of patients included in this study had experienced dyspnoea and oedema for nearly 24 hours prior to admission.[9]

Flexibility of care

As discussed in more detail in Chapter 3, home based intervention has proved to be the most consistent and effective strategy in reducing heart failure specific and all-cause hospital readmission, and hospital bed utilisation, in typically older heart failure patients.[4-6] This has also been our experience in the Glasgow service (see Chapter 6).

The service was originally set up to focus on home based intervention. However, increasing caseloads prompted us to explore methods of optimising the nurses' time management without compromising the quality of the service delivery. This has resulted in the development of nurse-led clinics at three of the hospital sites and for some of the patients this is the main form of contact they have with the service. The clinics operate with the same aims as the home based service but allow the nurses to see more patients in a shorter period of time. The clinics are based in hospital outpatient departments with access to cardiology investigations (for example ECG, blood tests, and advice from locally based cardiologists if required). Appointment times can be flexible. The clinic visit is followed up by a phone call to update the patient on any test results. Patients are made aware that the nurse is available by telephone if they experience any deterioration in symptoms or have any questions.

The clinic also simplifies the patient pathway to other services as the heart failure specialist nurse can facilitate referral to other health-care and social care professionals and investigations can be ordered without delay. If required, patients can be assured of an appointment within a few weeks of their last contact with the nurse. This can be an adjunct to medical cardiology or general medical outpatient clinics but increasingly patients are being discharged from these clinics with the understanding that they can be referred back if the heart failure nurse feels this is appropriate. This has the added benefit of reducing the numbers of patients attending other clinics and therefore reducing the waiting time for other patients.

Previous studies have identified that monitoring more stable heart failure patients at a dedicated heart failure clinic also reduces bed days and hospitalisation of these patients.[10,11] A recent study from Sweden found that patients who visit a nurse-led heart failure clinic after hospital discharge experience fewer adverse events and have a lower mortality than their peers who receive usual care.[12]

Service quality and monitoring

The Glasgow service is acknowledged as a United Kingdom leader and it is our intention to develop it in line with audit findings and feedback from clinicians and patients. At present the service is being monitored, evaluated, and audited at regular intervals. With co-ordinated training from an audit facilitator from the Health Authority the heart failure nurses have been trained in the use of the Microsoft Access database to retrieve pertinent data for audit purposes (see Chapter 6).

The database needs to be updated in order to record additional data on specific items such as palliative care and mortality, in addition to some suggested improvements for the audit programme. Existing medical and nursing guidelines are regularly reviewed and updated in line with current practice and technological advances. Information technology infrastructure is being developed in a way that will be of maximum benefit to staff (for example easy and rapid access to "results" systems such as echocardiography, haematology, and biochemistry). We hope to create a website which will be a useful tool for both patients and staff, whereby publications such as guidelines and annual reports could be posted, as well as providing a forum for useful information and contacts.

Providing a quality service: emerging issues

It would seem obvious that careful planning will not address all the issues and problems that arise when trying to introduce a completely new service. The following issues have either impinged on the effectiveness of the Glasgow service or required careful consideration and planning to maintain a quality service that evolves with each new challenge in heart failure.

Increasing workloads

Due to the nature of chronic heart failure, patients have to be managed and monitored on a long-term basis. Many patients in the service are unable to be discharged back to the original level of health care they were exposed to; there is no provision at present in the community to manage these high-risk patients. However, it is anticipated that the rollout of Glasgow's Chronic Disease Management Programme within community settings such as general practices and health centres will improve patient care in chronic heart disease and linking into this programme will be an effective way of managing these high-risk patients. It would be unrealistic to expect greatly increased survival rates for this cohort of patients since many are already NYHA Class III or IV. However, the impact of appropriate drug regimens and lifestyle education cannot be ignored as they are proving to be contributing factors towards lowering rates of morbidity and mortality. Thus the workload of the staff will continue to increase as more and more patients are exposed to the service.

The increasing workload, because of unanticipated follow-up requirements, has prompted the service to develop a formal discharge pathway for stable patients back to primary care services in Glasgow. The general practitioner is advised to check the patient's biochemistry in six months and the specialist heart failure nurses contact the practice nurse to ensure the patient is entered into the general practitioner's recall system. The patient and the general practitioner are advised to contact the service if there is clinical deterioration and the heart failure nurse will re-assess the patient.

Optimal use of resources

Using resources in different ways, for example ensuring adequate clerical help and ensuring expert nursing time is not used for tasks which can be performed by other staff, can offer the potential to increase patient numbers. Using telephone follow-up where possible and offering clinic access for routine blood monitoring for those able to travel are other possibilities to optimise resources. At present there are no additional resources available to further develop the service.

When further resources become available in the future we intend to expand the service to a wider group of heart failure patients. This will include providing education, support, and up-titration of therapy for newly diagnosed patients identified through open access echocardiography, as well as access for NYHA Class III and IV patients who have not had a hospital admission, and access for patients with heart failure with preserved left ventricular systolic function. The feedback received from primary care physicians has been positive; the only negative comments have been in relation to their inability to refer patients who have not had a hospital admission.

The service works closely with pharmacy colleagues who have also recently secured funding to carry out medication reviews in all Glasgow Health Authority Primary Care practices to identify patients with heart failure to start and/or optimise ACE inhibitor therapy. After the prevalent cases have been dealt with (late 2006) there will remain a system for dealing with newly diagnosed cases. The heart failure nurses and the pharmacy services would complement each other, with cross-referral between the heart failure nurse specialists and the pharmacists for ACE inhibitor initiation and up-titration.

The value of adding a pharmacist to the heart failure team has been demonstrated in the United States[13] but there is little published information and research about the value of pharmacists in such a role within the United Kingdom.[14]

Palliative care

In the Glasgow service, as in many parts of the United Kingdom, heart failure nurses have established formal links with palliative care services. At present there is minimal evidence available on which to base the management of the patient with end stage heart failure. This is obviously a very important issue that will require a multidisciplinary response and clear protocols (see Chapter 10).[15,16] The Glasgow Heart Failure Liaison Service hopes to be involved in the near future in a research study which will be carried out by a research fellow in palliative medicine. The objective of the study is to determine if liaison between specialist palliative care and clinical nurse specialists in heart failure improves symptom control, and quality of life for patients with NYHA Class 1V heart failure and their carers.

Exercise programmes

Until fairly recently it was thought that exercise was contra-indicated in patients with left ventricular systolic dysfunction, as it would result in impaired cardiac output and exacerbate underlying heart failure. In recent years, however, research suggests that structured, supervised aerobic and restrictive exercise programmes in carefully stratified patients can lead to a reduction in fatigue, an increase in functional class, and an overall improvement in sense of well being (see Chapter 8).[17] The inability to refer patients to such an exercise programme remains a gap in our service. At present only one site has a gym class dedicated to heart failure patients. At the time of publishing there are still ongoing discussions between the Heart Failure Liaison Service and established cardiac rehabilitation teams on how best to dovetail the care of this group of patients. The only avenue we have at present is to refer patients to local authority leisure classes (including phase 4 cardiac rehabilitation classes run by the British Association of Cardiac Rehabilitation trained leisure staff) through an exercise referral programme that runs in Glasgow. Many patients with chronic heart failure are not fit enough to take part in these classes and this naturally excludes a large proportion of our elderly population.

Links with academic institutions

Clinical nursing has perhaps traditionally been guilty of failing to forge strong links with academic institutions. In recent years there has been a culture shift and, in some specialties, clinical nurses have taken a more advanced role in working with academia. Since the service began most members of staff have had tentative links with educational facilities and organisations such as universities, the British Heart Foundation, and hospital staff. These links have been enhanced greatly in the past two years as a result of myself (as the service co-ordinator) being asked to design and run a nationally accredited educational programme. This programme, initially reserved for British Heart Foundation nurses, is now available to heart failure nurses throughout the United Kingdom. The key principles for training specialist heart failure nurses are described in Appendix 1.

Close educational relationships with these nurses involve our team members in providing teaching sessions at universities and actual clinical settings. It has also expanded, with the increased confidence and expertise of the specialist heart failure nurses speaking at national conferences. This has enabled the Glasgow service team to learn of, and gain exposure to, other models of care that provide clinic and home based intervention for this group of patients. Such cross-fertilisation is invaluable to all concerned. On a more local level the team at each hospital site provides educational talks to students and qualified staff, who also accompany the heart failure nurses on home visits.

Overview of the current status of the Glasgow service

There is considerable evidence in support of heart failure disease management programmes to prevent recurrent hospitalisation, stabilise and even decrease debilitating symptoms, and therefore improve quality of life in patients who suffer from chronic heart failure.[18] As described in more detail in Chapter 3, teams in both the Southern (Stewart *et al.* in Australia[19]) and Northern hemispheres (Strömberg *et al.* in Sweden[12]) have demonstrated that these programmes can also prolong the life of patients without compromising their quality of life.

A key component of the service in reducing hospital readmission may be the nurses' ability to adjust and optimise heart failure medications without medical consultation, and in accordance with agreed prescription guidelines (see Chapter 9). However it can also be argued that a more important component in reducing hospital readmission is continuity of care provided by the same healthcare professional. Previous research indicates that education and support are effective in improving patients' self-care behaviour; however, it is not enough to decrease readmission.[20] The Glasgow Heart Failure Liaison Service has all the components that are common to the most successful programmes of care in heart failure. These are listed below.

Key components of successful heart failure programmes of care

- Qualified specialist nurse who is able to work as an autonomous practitioner
- Provision of regular follow-up and assessment to detect early clinical deterioration
- Continued adjustment and optimisation of therapy according to agreed guidelines and protocols
- Close monitoring of blood chemistry
- Facilitation of self-management where possible
- Encouragement toward daily weight monitoring and to report any increase in weight of 1 kg or more per day which persists over more than 2–3 days
- Education – pharmacological and non-pharmacological
- Nursing support in order to facilitate communication and coordination of care between the patient and other healthcare professionals, including cardiologists and staff in the primary care setting
- Continued support for patients and their families/carers

The current literature also suggests that interventions involving a component of home based follow-up are more effective than those incorporating a clinic based follow-up alone. Similarly, a clinic based model appears to be more effective than strategies confined to the period of acute hospitalisation. Research undertaken by Ekman and colleagues in Sweden found that a clinic based approach was not suitable for all of their heart failure patients because of the time and effort taken to attend the clinic itself.[21] They therefore recommended a home based approach.

Our experience in the Glasgow service replicates the findings of the randomised controlled trials and current research in relation to the effectiveness of home based intervention. However, home based intervention is labour intensive and can be difficult to apply especially in rural areas. Specialist nurse-led interventions in heart failure must be adapted to the local healthcare environment. A model incorporating both clinic and home based intervention may ultimately be the most effective model in the light of finite healthcare resources, and the increasing role of interactive methods to monitor patients more closely has to be considered. As such, we will continue to monitor the effectiveness of the Glasgow service and introduce improvements/refinements as indicated to ensure that our primary aim, to improve the quality of life (and possibly end of life) of our patients and their carers, is achieved in the most cost-efficient manner.

References

1 Ashton CM. Care of patients with failing hearts: evidence for failures in clinical practice and health services research. *J Gen Intern Med* 1999;**14**:138–40.
2 Vinson JM, Rich MW, Sperry JC, Shah AS, McNamara T. Early readmission of elderly patients with congestive heart failure. *J Am Geriatr Soc* 1990;**38**:1290–5.
3 Chin MH, Goldman L. Factors contributing to the hospitalization of patients with congestive heart failure. *Am J Public Health* 1997;**87**:643–8.
4 Rich MW, Beckham V, Wittenberg C, Leven CL, Freedland KE, Carney RM. A multidisciplinary intervention to prevent the readmission of elderly patients with congestive heart failure. *N Engl J Med* 1995;**333**:1190–5.
5 Stewart S, Vandenbroek AJ, Pearson S, Horowitz JD. Prolonged beneficial effects of a home-based intervention on unplanned readmission and mortality among patients with congestive heart failure. *Arch Intern Med* 1999;**159**:257–61.
6 Blue L, Lang E, McMurray JJ, *et al*. Randomised controlled trial of specialist nurse intervention in heart failure. *BMJ* 2001;**323**:715–8.
7 Riegel B, Carlson B, Kopp Z, LePetri B, Glaser D, Unger A. Effect of a standardized nurse case management telephone intervention on resource use in patients with chronic heart failure. *Arch Intern Med* 2002;**162**: 705–12.
8 Erhardt L, Cline C. Heart failure clinics: a possible means of improving care. *Heart* 1998;**80**:428–9.
9 Michalsen A, Konig G, Thimme W. Preventable causative factors leading to hospital admission with decompensated heart failure. *Heart* 1998;**80**:427–41.
10 Cline CM, Israelsson BY, Willenheimer RB, Broms K, Erhardt LR. A cost effective management programme for heart failure reduces hospitalization. *Heart* 1998;**80**:442–6.
11 Doughty RN, Wright SP, Pearl A, *et al*. Randomized, controlled trial of integrated heart failure management: The Auckland Heart Failure Management Study. *Eur Heart J* 2002;**23**:139–46.
12 Strömberg A, Martensson J, Fridlund B, Levin LA, Karlsson JE, Dahlstrom U. Nurse-led heart failure clinics improve survival and self-care behaviour in patients with heart failure: results from a prospective, randomised trial. *Eur Heart J* 2003;**24**: 1014–23.
13 Gattis WA, Hasselblad V, Whellan DJ, O'Connor CM. Reduction in heart failure events by the addition of a clinical pharmacist to the heart failure management team: results of the Pharmacist in Heart Failure Assessment Recommendation and Monitoring (PHARM) Study. *Arch Intern Med* 1999;**159**:1939–45.
14 Lock J. The benefit of adding a pharmacist to the heart failure team. *Hospital Pharmacist* 2003;**10**:81–3.
15 Murray SA, Boyd K, Kendall M, *et al*. Dying of lung cancer or cardiac failure: prospective qualitative interview study of patients and their carers in the community. *BMJ* 2002;**325**:929–33.
16 Stewart S, McMurray JJ. Palliative care for heart failure? *BMJ* 2002;**325**:915–16.
17 Caldwell M, Dracup K. Team management of heart failure: The emerging role of exercise and implications for cardiac rehabilitation centers. *J Cardiopulm Rehabil* 2001;**21**:273–9.
18 Moser DK, Mann DL. Improving Outcomes in Heart Failure: It's not usual beyond usual care. *Circulation* 2002;**105**:2810–2.

19 Stewart S, Horowitz JD. Home-based intervention in congestive heart failure: long-term implications on readmission and survival. *Circulation* 2002;**105**: 2861–6.

20 Jaarsma T, Halfens R, Huijer Abu-Saad H, *et al*. Effects of education and support on self-care and resource utilization in patients with heart failure. *Eur Heart J* 1999; **20**:673–82.

21 Ekman I, Andersson B, Ehnfors M, Matejka B, Persson B, Fagerberg B. Feasibility of a nurse-monitored, outpatient-care programme for elderly patients with moderate-to-severe, chronic heart failure. *Eur Heart J* 1998;**19**:1254–60.

5: Establishing national heart failure services: can we afford not to?

SIMON STEWART

Introduction

As suggested by studies that describe the economic burden imposed by heart failure, and more specifically where the greatest expenditure occurs,[1-4] the key to cost-effectively managing the heart failure epidemic is to reduce hospital use – even at the expense of increasing levels of community based care and pharmacotherapy. Directly projecting the cost benefits of the programmes of care reviewed in Chapter 3 to the wider health care system without adjusting for additional expenses, however, would be too simplistic and over-estimate their potential cost benefits.[5] It is on the basis of these that we recently calculated the potential economic benefits from the creation of a UK-wide service designed to optimise the post-discharge management of more than 100 000 patients in the year 2000.[6]

Whilst the cost considerations and assumptions inherent in this analysis are not truly universal to other developed countries, the extent of potential cost savings relative to other "treatments" for heart failure (many of which are funded with a minimum of fuss despite their enormous cost!) means that the figures are extremely compelling. Moreover, as funding is a major limitation in applying these programmes of care, they provide a good framework for building a strong business case (local or national) for new or sustained funding of a fully functional heart failure service.

Economic benefits of applying a UK-wide heart failure service

As indicated above, directly projecting the potential cost impact of these programmes to the wider health care system without adjusting for additional expenses and a range of effects on healthcare utilisation rates would be too simplistic and over-estimate their potential cost benefits.[5] It is on this basis that we recently calculated the potential economic benefits of creating a UK-wide chronic heart failure (CHF) service based on a programme of nurse management.[6] Many of these data were derived from three of the key studies in Chapter 3, that described the benefits of nurse-led, home based interventions with a strong component of multidisciplinary involvement to optimise outcomes in older patients with CHF in the USA,[7] Australia,[8] and the UK.[9] More importantly, perhaps, a number of assumptions were modelled on the infrastructure and impact of the unique city-wide Glasgow Heart Failure Liaison Service in Scotland described in more detail in later chapters, and accurate UK data describing the burden and cost of CHF.[2,10] These data provided an accurate indication of the number and characteristics of CHF patients likely to be exposed to this service, the rate of recurrent hospitalisation, and the overall pattern and cost of health care following an acute hospitalisation.

Figure 5.1 summarises the basic structure and assumptions used to calculate the cost of creating a home based service, staffed by specialist heart failure nurses, in the UK. Based on the model of home based intervention applied as part of the city-wide Glasgow Heart Failure Liaison Service with the establishment of 60 distinct service areas, an appropriate workforce of specialist heart failure nurses and infrastructure support, we estimated that such a service would cost approximately £70 million per annum (year 2000 costs) to establish and maintain. This total cost takes into account the application of home visits and a substantial increase in pharmacotherapy, with the application of heart failure treatment closer to recommended guidelines[11] – applying gold standard treatment remains a universal but largely unachievable goal in optimising heart failure management.[12] Overall, the cost of establishing such a service would be equivalent to approximately 0·1% of total healthcare expenditure in the year 2000.[13] Based on observed rates of admission and readmission for chronic heart failure in the UK,[14,15] and clear guidelines for selecting suitable patients, a caseload of approximately 120 000 patients would be managed by this service.

During the year 2000, we estimate that approximately 47 000 of these patients would have normally accumulated around 594 000 days of recurrent hospital stay – representing an average of 12 days of readmission per patient. It should be noted that approximately 10% of these patients would experience multiple readmissions and accumulate a disproportionate number of hospital bed days relative to the remainder of the cohort. The total cost of these readmissions and associated bed utilisation to the UK National Health Service was estimated to be around £165 million (an average of £3500 per patient or 0·3% of the healthcare budget) with the need for post-discharge hospital care in surviving patients costing an additional £15 million during that year.[6]

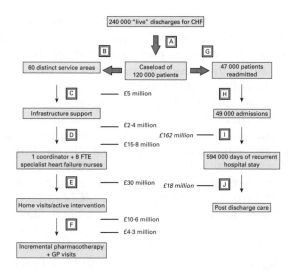

Figure 5.1 Patient caseload and cost assumptions used to estimate the cost of establishing a UK-wide specialist heart failure nurse service in the year 2000

A. We estimated that a total of 240 000 patients with CHF would be discharged alive from hospital in the UK in 2000. However, in accounting for the smaller proportion of patients who fulfil the following criteria: a) discharged to home, b) have documented evidence of left systolic ventricular dysfunction as opposed to diastolic dysfunction, c) over 65 years old and d) willing to be followed more closely, we conservatively assumed that only 50% of all CHF patients would receive incremental management.

B. The UK has approximately 60 million inhabitants and we assumed that a discrete team would service each million population in order to take into account variances within the population, in addition to the strengths and weaknesses of the local health care system.

C. We assumed that each service area (60 in total) would require establishment and ongoing infrastructure support (for example training and clerical costs) at a cost of £83 000 per annum.

D. We also assumed that each area would require a senior nurse coordinator (£40 000 per annum) and eight full-time equivalent nurses who would manage an average caseload of 200–250 patients per annum (based on estimated caseload) at a cost of £264 000 per annum for their salaries alone.

E. Each patient would receive an average of five home visits at a cost of £250 per annum for transport, equipment and investigative costs.

F. We assumed that the level of community health care would increase with an average of two additional general practitioner visits per patient emanating from the additional visits from the specialist heart failure nurses (at a cost of £36 per annum) and a marked increase (50%) in the cost of pharmacotherapy due to initiation and up-titration of treatment by the nurses (at a cost of £88 per annum).

G. Conversely, we estimated that approximately 47 000 of the approximately 120 000 patients who would be exposed to this service would normally be readmitted at least once during that year.

H. We also estimated that they would accumulate a total of 49 000 readmissions.

I. These readmissions would result in approximately 600 000 days of recurrent hospital stay (average of 12 days per patient) with an average cost of £3536 per readmitted patient.

J. We also assumed that each "live" discharge from a recurrent admission during that year would attract an average of two additional general practitioner visits and three outpatient clinic visits as part of standard post-discharge management.

Taking into account the combined "savings" of reduced bed utilisation and reduced levels of general practitioner and hospital outpatient consultations in the immediate post-discharge period,[2] we estimated that each 10% reduction in days of (all-cause) hospital bed utilisation in this cohort would result in a "cost saving" of £18 million in health care expenditure during the year 2000 in the UK.[6]

Based on all of these assumptions, Figure 5.2 shows the thresholds at which this theoretical UK-wide heart failure service might generate nominal savings equivalent to the cost of its implementation (£70 million per annum). As such, it shows that a 40% reduction in recurrent stay overall would generate savings approximately equivalent to the cost of running the service (£72 million per annum). Clearly, a 50% reduction in recurrent hospital stay (not totally unachievable given the likely benefits of reapplying the intervention in patients who survive a readmission and selection of higher risk patients during the recruitment phase) would generate significant cost savings (£169 000 per 1000 patients treated per annum or £42 000 per specialist heart failure nurse per annum). Alternatively, a 30% reduction in recurrent stay, whilst clinically important, would not be associated with any "savings". However, given the large expenditure of applying gold standard pharmacological treatment (approximately £10 million per annum) a cost that would normally be absorbed into the total healthcare budget, such a reduction would ensure that the service would remain economically attractive.

Based on the data present in Chapter 3 (Figure 3.3), it would appear that most chronic heart failure management programmes would be relatively cost-effective in this regard. Sensitivity analyses also confirmed that the service would remain economically attractive under a range of adverse conditions (i.e. increased application costs and reduced effect of recurrent hospital stay).[6] The fact that these interventions improve the quality of life of individuals with chronic heart failure[16,17] and, perhaps, prolong their life at the same time,[18] also needs to be considered.

It is important to note that the economic benefits of applying better management of heart failure can extend beyond the short term – i.e. accumulative costs will not be shifted to the healthcare budget in subsequent years. Figure 5.3 shows the accumulative effect of a single specialist heart failure nurse on recurrent readmissions based on a case load of 300 patients per annum. These data are derived from recently presented data emanating from a home based intervention in Adelaide, South Australia.[19]

Comparisons with "other" heart failure treatments

How do these data compare to similar analyses of pharmacological agents used to treat chronic heart failure? It should be noted firstly that

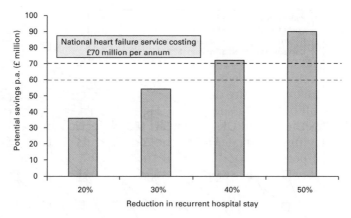

Figure 5.2 Economic impact of a UK-wide, specialist nurse heart failure service

very rarely do treatment options save money (the phenomenon of shifting costs beyond the horizon of study follow-up being a classic caveat in interpreting this type of data).[3,4,20] Regardless of this important issue, it would appear that the heart failure service compares favourably to other therapeutic options in heart failure. For example, the cost of applying the service on a UK-wide basis to 120 000 patients was estimated to be approximately £500 per patient without the additional cost of pharmacotherapy.[6] Alternatively, based on a 40% reduction in recurrent hospital stay, it was estimated that savings equivalent to £600 per patient (a 20% reduction in costs relative to its initial application) would be generated during the year 2000. A recent pharmacoeconomic analysis of the COPERNICUS study applied to the UK,[21] utilising the same underlying data and assumptions, showed that the cost of applying carvedilol in similar patients with moderate to severe chronic heart failure would be around £550 per patient and produce savings equivalent to £661 per patient treated (also a 20% reduction in costs relative to its initial application). As the COPERNICUS data[21] were consistent with those generated from CIBIS II economic data,[22] it is tempting to conclude that a heart failure service would be as cost-effective as β-blockers in treating heart failure. Moreover, given the evidence in non-selected patients who are generally older and with greater comorbidity than those patients enrolled in clinical trials,[23,24] it might be safe to assume that this service would be easier to apply and offer in a more effective manner than many new therapeutic agents. It would also assist the introduction of new therapeutic strategies into the wider heart failure population. Certainly, a coordinated approach to applying best practice in managing heart failure, both in terms of pharmacological treatments, and in terms of the type of supportive strategies that will facilitate their application and have additional benefits, is required.

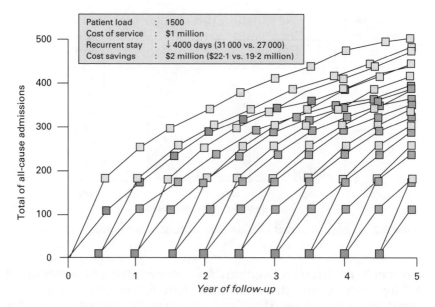

Figure 5.3 Accumulative impact of a specialist heart failure nurse on recurrent hospital readmissions over five years

The "matrix" of squares represents accumulated admissions on the basis of exposure (dark squares) versus non-exposure (usual care – light squares) to a home based intervention. Over a five-year period the specialist nurse manages 1500 patients in various stages of their natural history with the greatest impact occurring within six months of their "index admission". Based on complete follow-up of heart failure patients over a five-year period,[19] these data show that a single specialist heart failure nurse would generate significant cost savings over a prolonged period.

Conclusions

The data supporting the widespread introduction of services based on the expert management applied by specialist heart failure nurses are compelling – both on the basis of individual benefits to the patient and their caregivers (as described in more detail in Chapter 3), and on a financial basis. National heart failure services based on the expertise of specialist heart failure nurses have the potential to deliver significant cost savings and enable the incumbent healthcare system to operate more efficiently.

Unfortunately, while there are often clear pathways to facilitate the rapid introduction of effective pharmacological agents used to treat heart failure, funding for the type of cost-effective heart failure service described in this chapter is sub-optimal in many developed countries.

The compelling data presented in this chapter provide a sound basis for deriving both local and national business plans for the establishment and continued application of this type of intervention.

References

1 McMurray JJV, Hart W, Rhodes G. An evaluation of the cost of heart failure to the National Health Service in the UK. *Br J Med Econ* 1993;6:91–8.
2 Stewart S, Jenkins A, Buchan S, McGuire A, Capewell S, McMurray JJ. The current cost of heart failure to the National Health Service in the UK. *Eur J Heart Fail* 2002;4:361–71.
3 Mark DB. Economics of treating heart failure. *Am J Cardiol* 1997;80:33H–38H.
4 Weintraub WS, Cole J, Tooley JF. Cost and cost-effectiveness studies in heart failure research. *Am Heart J* 2002;143:565–76.
5 Stewart S, Horowitz JD. Specialist nurse management programmes: economic benefits in the management of heart failure *Pharmacoeconomics* 2003;21:225–40.
6 Stewart S, Blue L, Walker A, Morrison C, McMurray JJ. An economic analysis of specialist heart failure nurse management in the UK: can we afford not to implement it? *Eur Heart J* 2002;23:1369–78.
7 Rich MW, Beckham V, Wittenberg C, Leven CL, Freedland KE, Carney RM. A multidisciplinary intervention to prevent the readmission of elderly patients with congestive heart failure. *N Engl J Med* 1995;333:1190–5.
8 Stewart S, Marley JE, Horowitz JD. Effects of a multidisciplinary, home-based intervention on unplanned readmissions and survival among patients with chronic congestive heart failure: a randomised controlled study. *Lancet* 1999;354: 1077–83.
9 Blue L, Lang E, McMurray JJ, *et al*. Randomised controlled trial of specialist nurse intervention in heart failure. *BMJ* 2001;323:715–18.
10 Stewart S, MacIntyre K, Capewell S, McMurray JJV. Heart failure and the aging population: an increasing burden in the 21st Century? *Heart*. 2003;89:49–53.
11 Remme WJ, Swedberg K. Guidelines for the diagnosis and treatment of chronic heart failure. *Eur Heart J* 2001;22:1527–60.
12 Clarke KW, Gray D, Hampton JR. Evidence of inadequate investigation and treatment of patients with heart failure. *Br Heart J* 1994;71:584–7.
13 UK National Health Service (2000) (Accessed July 2002): http://www.doh.gov.uk/nhsexec/refcosts/2000
14 Stewart S, MacIntyre K, MacLeod MMC, Bailey AEM, Capewell S, McMurray JJ. Trends in hospitalization for heart failure in Scotland, 1990–1996. An epidemic that has reached its peak? *Eur Heart J* 2001;22:209–17.
15 Stewart S, Demers C, Murdoch DR, *et al*. Substantial between-hospital variation in outcome following first emergency admission for heart failure. *Eur Heart J* 2002;23: 650–7.
16 McMurray JJ, Stewart S. Nurse-led multidisciplinary intervention in chronic heart failure. *Heart* 1998;80:430–1.
17 Rich MW. Heart failure disease management: a critical review. *J Cardiac Fail* 1999;5:64–75.
18 Stewart S, Berry C, McMurray JJV. Multidisciplinary intervention in congestive heart failure – does it reduce morbidity and mortality? *Eur Heart J* 2003;24:65.
19 Stewart S. Modulating the cost of prolonged survival in heart failure: long-term benefits of a nurse-led, multidisciplinary, home-based intervention. *J Cardiac Fail* 2003;5:S5.
20 Rich MW, Nease RF.Cost-effectiveness analysis in clinical practice: the case of heart failure. *Arch Intern Med* 1999;159:1690–700.
21 CIBIS-II Investigators and Health Economics Group. Reduced costs with bisoprolol treatment for heart failure: An economic analysis of the second Cardiac Insufficiency Bisoprolol Study (CIBIS-II). *Eur Heart J* 2001;22:1021–31.

22 Stewart S, McMurray JJV, Hebborn A, Coats AJS, Packer M for the COPERNICUS Study Group. Carvedilol reduces the cost of medical care in severe heart failure: an economic analysis of the COPERNICUS Study applied to the United Kingdom. *Circulation* 2001;**104**(Suppl II):717.

23 Petrie MC, Dawson NF, Murdoch DR, Davie AP, McMurray JJ. Failure of women's hearts. *Circulation* 1999;**99**:2334–41.

24 Petrie MC, Berry C, Stewart S, McMurray JJ. Failing ageing hearts. *Eur Heart J* 2001; **22**:1978–90.

Section 3:
From theory to practice

6: A blueprint for identifying and managing patients within a heart failure service

KIRSTIN RUSSELL, ALISON FREEMAN,
LYNDA BLUE, SIMON STEWART

Introduction

As discussed in Chapter 4, the process of translating research into practice is not an easy one. In establishing the Glasgow Heart Failure Liaison Service many people have dedicated an enormous amount of time and energy to ensure that this service can be replicated and maintained as the number of collaborating hospitals, specialist heart failure nurses, health care professionals, and miscellaneous organisations grows. The ultimate aim, of course, is to ensure that the quality of service provided to patients is consistently maintained at the highest possible standard over a prolonged period, irrespective of its location and the individuals involved. It is within this context that this chapter presents the pivotal protocols, materials, and datasets that have been established to ensure that the reputation and impact of the Glasgow service is safeguarded.

The Glasgow Heart Failure Liaison Service in operation

The following sections present, in logical order, the protocols used to identify and manage patients within the Glasgow service. These can be easily implemented elsewhere to establish the framework for a similar service. As described in the first edition of this book, it is essential to identify the key stakeholders in the management of heart failure and establish clear and constructive lines of communication to ensure that the following protocols can be adapted and refined to best suit the local healthcare environment.

Screening and recruitment

In order to select appropriate patients to be managed in an evidence-based manner, strict inclusion criteria have to be utilised. Patients need to be identified without delay while in hospital and this requires that the multidisciplinary team involved in their care is aware of the existence of the heart failure service and how to access it. They must also be aware of the inclusion and exclusion criteria to avoid inappropriate patients being referred.

Inclusion criteria

All patients who have had an emergency hospital admission related to worsening heart failure. The underlying syndrome of chronic heart failure must be caused by left ventricular systolic dysfunction (determined by echocardiography, radionuclide ventriculography, or coronary angiography).

NB. In light of the current interest in those with chronic heart failure associated with preserved left ventricular systolic function (so called diastolic heart failure) and the potential for improving outcomes in such patients (see Chapter 2), if appropriate resources and expertise are available, there is no reason why such patients cannot be included for active intervention. In Glasgow, there has been a conscious effort to establish the service before addressing the issues (for example resources and specific treatment protocols required to effectively manage this additional cohort of patients).

Exclusion criteria

- Unwilling to have this support.
- Unable to participate in the service due to living alone and having:
  - impaired cognitive ability determined by the abbreviated mental test
  - major communication problems.
- Other immediately life threatening illness (for example advanced malignancy).
- Living outside the institutional/health authority geographic area of responsibility.
- Discharged to long-term care (at present patients discharged to long-term nursing care are excluded; a proposed service development may include these patients).
- Attending day hospital facilities on a regular basis for medical management (for example a pre-established heart failure clinic that would obviate the need for additional management).
- Patient history of abusive behaviour towards healthcare professionals.

NHS

Greater
Glasgow

**GREATER GLASGOW
PRIMARY CARE
NHS TRUST**

Heart Failure
Liaison Service

Please refer in-patients presenting with dyspnoea and/or peripheral oedema secondary to left ventricular systolic dysfunction, for post-discharge follow-up to:

Sister ****** *******

Ext: ****

If no reply, please leave contact details on the answering machine.

Figure 6.1 Poster for display in hospital wards

If a patient does not strictly meet the inclusion criteria but they may still potentially benefit from more intensive management, their possible recruitment to the service should be discussed with colleagues or the nurse coordinator. If necessary the designated cardiologist responsible for the overall management of patients being recruited from the particular institution should also be consulted.

Patients are recruited from general medical and cardiology wards. Information about the service is clearly displayed in each of these areas. Due to the high turnover of junior medical staff it is important to raise the profile of the service on a regular basis to avoid appropriate patients being missed. Key strategies in this regard are:

- educational talks to nursing staff
- presentations at grand rounds
- regular visits to the wards.

An A3 laminated poster (see Figure 6.1) is displayed in all medical, cardiology, and care of the elderly wards in participating hospitals in Glasgow.

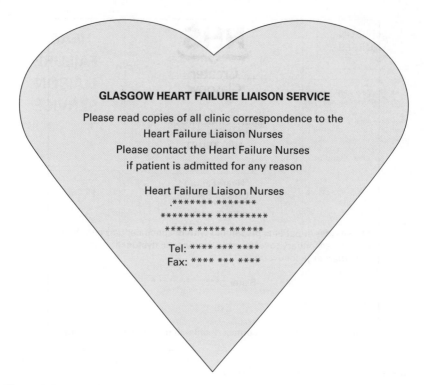

GLASGOW HEART FAILURE LIAISON SERVICE

Please read copies of all clinic correspondence to the
Heart Failure Liaison Nurses
Please contact the Heart Failure Nurses
if patient is admitted for any reason

Heart Failure Liaison Nurses
.******* *******
********* *********
***** ***** ******

Tel: **** *** ****
Fax: **** *** ****

Figure 6.2   Service identification label

Service identification labels are attached to the front of hospital case notes when patients are recruited (see Figure 6.2). This label asks that the service be contacted should the patient be readmitted and that copies of all clinic letters are sent to the responsible heart failure nurse.

If patients are not referred during their hospital admission the patient's general practitioner (primary care physician) can still refer them to the service on a post-discharge basis. Local general practitioners, therefore, must be made aware of this additional pathway to the service and encouraged to use it whenever patients are inappropriately missed during the hospital screening process. Figure 6.3 shows the type of information leaflet that is also available in each ward and distributed to primary care colleagues to ensure that few, if any, eligible patients are missed by the screening process as awareness of the service grows.

A pilot questionnaire (see Figure 6.4) has also been sent to nurses working with general practitioners in the East End of Glasgow. The aim of this is to gauge the level of knowledge and awareness about the service in this important group of nurses. The plan is to extend the pilot to other areas of the city.

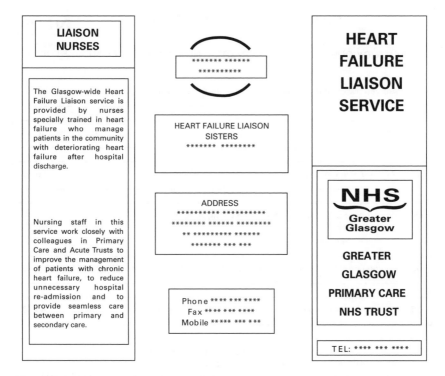

Figure 6.3 Service information leaflet

Having identified patients who meet the inclusion criteria, agreed nursing guidelines are then implemented in respect of baseline information being documented and appropriate measures set in place to ensure follow-up after discharge.

Guidelines and protocols

Comprehensive nursing and medical therapy guidelines have been formulated to ensure the effective management of patients recruited to the Glasgow service. Some of the areas covered by these include:

Nursing guidelines

- signs and symptoms
- home based assessment
- monitoring
- non-pharmacological management
- investigations in relation to heart failure.

HEART FAILURE LIAISON SERVICE

PILOT STUDY QUESTIONNAIRE – PRACTICE NURSE INVOLVEMENT

Q1. Are you aware of the existence of the Heart Failure Service? Yes ☐ No ☐

Q2. Do you know how to access the HF Service? Yes ☐ No ☐

Q3. Are you aware of the objectives of the HF Service ? Yes ☐ No ☐

Q4. Do you have any patients who are receiving support from the HF Service ? Yes ☐ No ☐

Q5. Do you currently receive any communication from the HF Nurses? Yes ☐ No ☐

Q6. Would you like more communication with the HF Nurses? Yes ☐ No ☐

Q7. If you see a patient who is receiving the support of the HF Service and you notice a deterioration in their heart failure symptoms, would you contact the Heart Failure Nurses? Yes ☐ No ☐

Q8. If you were checking a patient's blood for any reason, would you let the Heart Failure Nurses know this and inform them of the result? Yes ☐ No ☐

Q9. If patients were to be discharged from the HF Service back to standard care in the community, would you be willing to monitor their progress on a six monthly basis (this would involve a U&Es check as a method of measuring tolerance to ACE inhibitor therapy)? Yes ☐ No ☐

Q10. Would you be interested in learning more about current best practice in the local management of heart failure? Yes ☐ No ☐

Please use this space to record any additional comments you may have

Many thanks for taking the time to complete this questionnaire

Figure 6.4 Questionnaire for practice nurses

Medical therapy guidelines

Medical therapy guidelines include drug therapy and blood chemistry monitoring protocols for the following types of drugs:

- loop diuretics
- thiazide diuretics and metolazone
- angiotensin converting enzyme inhibitors and angiotensin receptor blockers
- β-blockers
- spironolactone
- digoxin
- non-heart failure specific pharmacotherapy.

Both the nursing (Chapters 7 and 8) and medical therapy (Chapter 9) management of heart failure are discussed in greater detail in subsequent chapters and are supported by a number of case studies highlighting common clinical issues arising from such management (Appendix 2).

Enrolment to the service

The information collected when recruiting eligible patients to the service consists of demographic profile, past medical history, medication prior to admission and on discharge, allergies and drug intolerances, cardiovascular status, ECG and echocardiographic results (if there is no indication of left ventricular assessment in the case notes the heart failure nurse can request an echocardiogram for clarification), blood chemistry, and full blood count (see enrolment form: Figure 6.5).

Once these data are collected they are transferred onto the service database where all further contact with the patient is also recorded. Future plans for data collection in Glasgow include changing to a paperless system, the Greater Glasgow NHS IT Strategy. This will allow access to all data from both clinics and home visits. It will also be possible to access data from general practitioner surgeries, with appropriate security.

Individualised patient follow-up

One of the key aims of post-discharge follow-up is to provide tailored management to meet the individual's needs in accordance with the service's nursing and medical therapy guidelines. Ultimately, the specialist heart failure nurse is responsible for the following:

- continued adjustment and optimisation of medical therapy where indicated according to established guidelines
- monitoring the patient's blood chemistry and clinical status closely, particularly if there is evidence of biochemical instability and deteriorating symptoms, or if changes to the medication regimen have been made (monitoring as per medical therapy protocol).

| Heart Failure Liaison Service
Enrolment Form | Form EF1 |

DEMOGRAPHICS

Patient Name ....   Marital status (specify) ....

Hospital No ....   CHI No .... Next of Kin ....

Date of Birth .... Sex M / F   Relationship(specify) ....

Address ....   Address ....

Postcode ....   Postcode ....

Telephone ....   Telephone ....

Ethnic Origin   White ☐ Black Caribbean ☐ Black African ☐ Black Other ☐

           Indian ☐ Pakistani ☐ Bangladeshi ☐ Chinese ☐ Other ....

GP ....   **Social Circumstances**

GP Address ....   Lives With (specify): ....

           District nurse   N ☐   Y ☐ Frequency ....

           Home Help   N ☐   Y ☐ Frequency ....

Postcode ....   Meals/Wheels   N ☐   Y ☐ Frequency ....

Telephone ....   Day Care   N ☐   Y ☐ Frequency ....

Practice No ....

Discharge arrangements

Discharge date ....   Date of first visit ....

Destination: Home ☐   Other ☐   Specify ....

Follow-up clinic date and consultant:

Comments:

Allergies:

Notes: ....

....

....

....

....

....

....

Review date October 2001   Copyright Greater Glasgow Primary Care NHS Trust

Figure 6.5   Service enrolment form

Heart Failure Liaison Service Enrolment Form	Form EF1

BASELINE PAST MEDICAL HISTORY & RISK FACTORS

Cause of CHF Ischaemic ☐ Valvular ☐

Cardiomyopathy ☐ Hypertensive ☐

Other ....

Chr Renal F	N ☐ Y ☐	
IHD	N ☐ Y ☐	
COPD	N ☐ Y ☐	
Asthma	N ☐ Y ☐	
CVA/TIA	N ☐ Y ☐	
PVD	N ☐ Y ☐	
MI	N ☐ Y ☐	Date ....
MI Site	....	
Angiogram	N ☐ Y ☐	Date ....
PTCA	N ☐ Y ☐	Date ....
CABG	N ☐ Y ☐	Date ....
Angina	N ☐ Y ☐	

Raised Lipids	N ☐ Y ☐
Hypertension	N ☐ Y ☐
Alcohol XS	N ☐ Former ☐ Current ☐
Overweight	N ☐ Y ☐
Smoker	N ☐ Former ☐ Current ☐
Diabetes	N ☐ Y ☐
Diabetic Therapy	....
Rh Fever	N ☐ Y ☐
Valve Disease	N ☐ Y ☐
Prosthetic Valves	....
Date of last op	....
AF/Flutter	N ☐ Y ☐
Cardiac Arrest	N ☐ Y ☐
Pacemaker	N ☐ Y ☐
Drug Intolerance	....

Drugs on Admission

NAME	DOSE	FREQUENCY

Review date October 2001   Copyright Greater Glasgow Primary Care NHS Trust

Figure 6.5 continued

Heart Failure Liaison Service
Enrolment Form

Form EF1

ASSESSMENT ON WARD

Admitted	Precipitating Cause Unstable Angina ☐ MI ☐
Date of visit	For Admission Chest Infection ☐ Arrhythmia ☐
Discharged	Social Admission ☐ Anaemia ☐
Hospital .... Ward	Medication Change ☐ Thyroid ☐
Consultant	Drug Compliance ☐ Alcohol XS ☐
	Other (specify) ....

Status at Discharge

NYHA N☐ I☐ II☐ III☐ IV☐   HR .... bpm Weight .... kg BMI........ Height ....

Fatigue N☐ Y☐ ....Rhythm Sinus ☐ AF☐ Paced ☐ Other

Dizziness N☐ Y☐ ....BP .... /........ mmHg (......./...... mmHg standing)

Palpitations N☐ Y☐ ....Oedema N☐ Ankle ☐ Calf ☐ Thigh ☐ Waist ☐

Angina N☐ I☐ II☐ III☐ IV☐ Ascites N☐ Mild ☐ Moderate ☐ Severe ☐

JVP N☐ Raised ☐ Markedly Raised ☐

Questionnaire score: Creps N☐ Few ☐ Basal ☐ Mid-chest ☐ Widespread

LWHF ....

Drugs on Discharge

		NAME	DOSE	FREQUENCY
Loop Diuretic				
Thiazide/Metolazone				
Spironolactone				
ACE / ATII				
Beta-blocker				
Digoxin				
GTN spray				
Nitrate				
Ca⁺⁺ Blocker				
Aspirin				
Warfarin				
Other Medication	1			
	2			
	3			
	4			
	5			

Medication started, but not continued

NAME	DOSE	FREQUENCY	REASON

Review date October 2001   Copyright Greater Glasgow Primary Care NHS Trust

Figure 6.5   continued

Heart Failure Liaison Service **Enrolment Form**	Form EF1

PRE-DISCHARGE TESTS

ECG

Date .... Copy obtained N □ Y □

Rhythm   Sinus □ AF □ Paced □ Other ....

LVH   N □ Y □

Conduction   1° HB □ LBBB □ RBBB □

Old MI   ....

LV Function / Valve Assessment

Modality   Echo □ RNVG □ Cath □   Date ....

Ejection fraction   .... %

LV Dysfunction   Mild □ Mild/Mod □ Mod □ Mod/Severe □ Severe □

Mitral Stenosis   None □ Mild □ Mild/Mod □ Mod □ Mod/Severe □ Severe □

Aortic Stenosis   None □ Mild □ Mild/Mod □ Mod □ Mod/Severe □ Severe □

Mitral Regurgitation   None □ Mild □ Mild/Mod □ Mod □ Mod/Severe □ Severe □

Aortic Regurgitation   None □ Mild □ Mild/Mod □ Mod □ Mod/Severe □ Severe □

Tricuspid Regurgitation   None □ Mild □ Mild/Mod □ Mod □ Mod/Severe □ Severe □

LV Hypertrophy   N □ Y □

Blood Tests

Date	Date	Date ....
Na .... mmol/l	Hb .... g/dl	Other ....
K .... mmol/l	WCC .... $\times 10^9$/l	....
Cl .... mmol/l	Platelets .... $\times 10^9$/l	....
Bic .... mmol/l		
Urea .... mmol/l		
Creatinine .... umol/l		
Glucose .... mmol/l		

Comments:

Nurse's Signature: _____   **Date:** _____

Nurse's Name: _____

Review date October 2001   Copyright Greater Glasgow Primary Care NHS Trust

Figure 6.5 continued

Assessment criteria and schedule of follow-up nurse contact

Minimum intervention

Regardless of their risk profile, all patients (and their families and carers where appropriate) enrolled in the Glasgow service are offered the following:

- a home visit within one week of hospital discharge to assess them in the home environment
- a second home visit one to four weeks after hospital discharge
- a phone call at three months (substituted with home visit if no telephone)
- access to the service if they are readmitted to hospital.

Incremental intervention according to individuals needs

Based on the following three components of assessment, patients also receive a more prolonged and intensive programme of follow-up:

1. Symptomatic status
   Patients can be (arbitrarily) divided into those who are symptom-free and those in whom symptoms persist following hospital discharge. In both of these groups there will be patients who are either at "low" or at "high" risk for future events such as unplanned readmission or even death without hospitalisation.
2. Appropriateness of treatment
   Regardless of an individual's symptoms, treatment will be either *appropriate* or *inappropriate*.
3. Risk status
   Patients can be considered to be at either high or low risk of future events on the following basis.

Low-risk patients are:

- knowledgeable about their condition and treatment
- compliant with medication and diet
- receiving adequate social support
- not in need of changes.

High-risk patients have:

- a poor understanding of their condition and its treatment
- a history of recurrent admissions for heart failure
- poor compliance with medication and diet
- inadequate social support
- an unsuitable lifestyle.

It should be noted that these are principles of assessment only and that ultimately it is the expert judgement of the specialist heart failure nurse, in conjunction with the advice of the other healthcare professionals and the availability of resources (i.e. by considering current caseload demands) that determines the duration and intensity of follow-up. However, using the above criteria, it is possible to roughly categorise the needs of patients using the following groups and the intensity and frequency of care can be modulated accordingly.

Group 1 patients: found to be symptom free at the first home visit

(a) Low risk and appropriately treated For patients at low risk and appropriately treated, regular home visiting is unlikely to have much benefit and telephone contact on an infrequent basis (for example, three monthly) is all that is required. These patients will be encouraged to make non-scheduled telephone contact should their condition deteriorate. These patients will therefore receive the "minimum service" unless their condition or risk profile subsequently changes.

(b) Low risk but inappropriately treated In this group of patients the main aim is to optimise the patient's medication in accordance with the agreed medication and nursing guidelines. Patients may be visited weekly until the medication regimen is appropriate and their blood chemistry is stable. Regular telephone contact is maintained until the patient is clinically stable. These patients are encouraged to make non-scheduled telephone contact should their condition deteriorate.

(c) High risk but appropriately treated In high-risk, appropriately treated patients, intervention is aimed at improving the patient's understanding of the condition and its treatment, and where indicated increasing social support. The patient may be visited weekly until modifiable risk factors are fully addressed, in accordance with the patient's needs and wishes. Regular telephone calls may also be required until all modifiable issues are addressed. Patients will also be encouraged to make non-scheduled telephone contact should their condition deteriorate.

(d) High risk and inappropriately treated The intervention in this group is aimed at improving the patient's understanding of the condition and its treatment; where indicated, increasing social support; and optimising the patient's medication in accordance with the agreed medical therapy guidelines (monitoring medication changes and blood chemistry). Home visits may be undertaken on a weekly basis until the patient is compliant with an appropriate medication regimen and modifiable risk factors have been fully

addressed, in accordance with the patient's needs and wishes. Regular telephone calls may also be required until all modifiable issues are addressed. Patients will also be encouraged to make non-scheduled telephone contact should their condition deteriorate.

Group 2 Patients: found to be symptomatic or clinically unstable at the first home visit

(a) Low risk and appropriately treated One of the objectives of specialist nurse intervention in low-risk appropriately treated patients is, where possible, to adjust what is already considered to be appropriate therapy to improve the patient's clinical status and to minimise any adverse effects of treatment. This will involve application of the medication guidelines and appropriate monitoring of any therapeutic changes implemented (including blood chemistry). The patient *may* require a number of home visits if there is scope for symptoms to improve. *It must be acknowledged, however, that it may not be possible to resolve symptoms completely in all patients and therefore further adjustment of treatment may be inappropriate.* However, the patient is also likely to benefit from other components of this type of intervention. The second objective, therefore, is to provide additional support to individuals who remain symptomatic despite optimal therapy but who would, for example, benefit from psychological and/or, ultimately, palliative care support. On this basis, further home visits may be warranted, followed by regular telephone follow-up thereafter. Patients will also be encouraged to make non-scheduled telephone contact should their condition deteriorate.

(b) Low risk but inappropriately treated The purpose of the intervention in this group of patients is to adjust their therapy to improve clinical status and minimise adverse effects, by application of the medication guidelines and appropriate monitoring of any therapeutic changes implemented (including blood chemistry). Patients will require home visits until symptoms improve and the patient is compliant with an appropriate regimen. Regular telephone calls may be required until appropriate therapy or clinical stability is achieved. *It may not be possible to resolve symptoms completely in all patients even after appropriate treatment is implemented.* Patients will also be encouraged to make non-scheduled telephone contact should their condition deteriorate.

(c) High risk but appropriately treated The object of intervention in high-risk patients who are appropriately treated is to adjust therapy to improve symptoms and signs and to minimise the potential for adverse effects. This will involve application of medication guidelines

and appropriate monitoring of any therapeutic changes implemented (including blood chemistry). Patients may require home visits until symptoms have improved and risk factors are fully addressed in accordance with the patient's needs and wishes. Regular telephone contact should be maintained until all important issues are addressed. *It may not be possible to resolve symptoms completely in all patients.* Patients will also be encouraged to make non-scheduled telephone contact should their condition deteriorate.

(d) High risk and inappropriately treated The object of intervention in inappropriately treated high-risk patients is to adjust therapy to improve the patient's clinical status and minimise any adverse effects of treatment, by application of the medication guidelines and appropriate monitoring of any therapeutic changes implemented (including blood chemistry). Patients may require weekly home visits until they are compliant with an appropriate medication regimen, their symptoms have improved, and modifiable risk factors have been fully addressed in accordance with the patient's needs and wishes. Regular telephone contact should be maintained until all important issues are addressed. *Once again, it should be remembered that it may not be possible to resolve symptoms completely in all patients.* Patients will also be encouraged to make non-scheduled telephone contact should their condition deteriorate.

Summary of the pattern of specialist nurse intervention

Table 6.1 is a theoretical schedule of home-based intervention based on the above groups. It should be noted that clinic based visits can be substituted for home visits and that the same principles for altering the frequency and intensity of the intervention based on the patient profile and immediate needs apply if a clinic based approach is adopted.

Documenting and tracking patient management

It should come as no surprise that is often hard to keep track of the complex and difficult process that is managing patients with chronic heart failure. Documenting patient details and tracking changes in their clinical status and treatment is, however, an important task that facilitates an overall understanding of each individual case. There are many commercially available database systems used to track patients with heart failure. However, the Glasgow service uses a comprehensive heart failure specific database that was specially designed (in Glasgow) and implemented to facilitate the activities of the service. The database, called ATHENA, is now being widely used across the UK.

Table 6.1 Scheme for applying a specialist nurse-led service in heart failure*

	Group 1 (symptom-free)				Group 2 (symptomatic)			
	A	B	C	D	A	B	C	D
Initial home visit within 1 week	✓	✓	✓	✓	✓	✓	✓	✓
Second home visit at 1–2 weeks	✓	✓	✓	✓	✓	✓	✓	✓
Routine 3-monthly phone-calls	✓	✓	✓	✓	✓	✓	✓	✓
Weekly home visits for the first month		✓	✓	✓	✓	✓	✓	✓
Weekly home visits extended for 1–2 months								✓
Weekly phone calls to reassess status				✓		✓	✓	✓
Monthly phone call to reassess health status			✓		✓			
Re-application of service if readmitted	✓	✓	✓	✓	✓	✓	✓	✓

*Columns A, B, C, and D refer to the four groups described on pages 107–9: A = low risk, appropriately treated; B = low risk inappropriately treated; C = high risk, appropriately treated; D = high risk, inappropriately treated.

Key points

All patients subject to a "safety-net" of at least two home visits plus 3-monthly phone calls.

Patients regularly reassessed and the amount of follow-up increased or reduced based on their clinical and psychosocial status.

The specialist heart failure nurse's aim is to maximise the impact of initial intervention and limit contact thereafter (excepting patient-initiated phone calls).

The management of patients who are either symptomatic or receiving inappropriate treatment after 3 months should be subject to review (for example by the specialist heart failure nurse coordinator in consultation with the cardiologist and general practitioner).

The use of this database allows for the collection and analysis of a vast amount of data and it can be used in conjunction with outpatient clinic visits or as part of a nurse-led liaison service between hospitals and general practitioners.

The programme provides the following functions:

- recording of patient contacts concerning:
  - admissions to hospital
  - doctor-led heart failure clinics
  - nurse-led heart failure clinics

- home visits
- telephone calls
- general practice visits.

The information recorded includes signs, symptoms, cardiac tests, blood tests, medication, etc. This provides an electronic patient record.

- generation of letters to:
  - the patient
  - the patient's general practitioner
  - local general practitioner emergency medical services
  - palliative care services
  - transplant services
  - social workers
  - others, for example consultant referrals.

The letters generated are structured in accordance with good communication guidelines.

- scheduling of planned visits
- to-do list and diary entries.

ATHENA stores all the information required to meet the National Service Framework for Coronary Heart Disease in the UK. It also provides audit facilities in line with the National Service Framework guidelines (see below) and has been designed to allow many users to access the same patient information from different computers. However, this means that the computers all have to be linked together to be able to share this information. The Glasgow service has desktop PCs installed in the nurses' office with the patient data held on a hospital server computer. Each computer is attached to the hospital network. This has many advantages – the patient data are secure and backed up. When the nurses go out on visits, they print off the patient's details – this can either be the last letter or a special summary sheet. They jot down their findings in the patient's home and when they get back to the hospital they enter this into ATHENA. They can then print off letters to the general practitioner or other colleagues regarding that visit. This system works very well – the Glasgow nurses have performed many thousand visits each over the last few years. Figures 6.6 and 6.7 show snapshots from the dataset and a typical letter generated from collated information, which illustrate its usefulness in facilitating patient management.

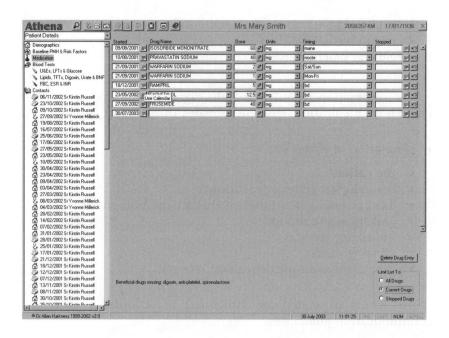

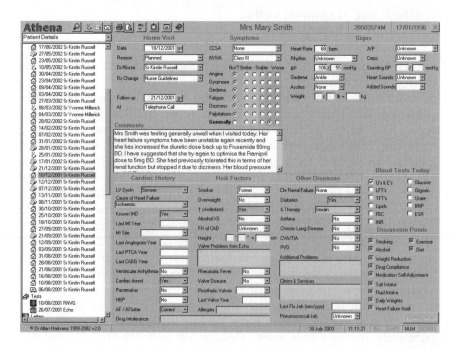

Figure 6.6 Typical ATHENA dataset

Maintaining high standards: audit data from the service

As noted above, the ATHENA dataset is an important source of information on both an individual and a service level. The latter is evidenced by the wealth of information, some of which is presented below in respect to the overall activity of the Glasgow service. As described in the first edition of this book, it is extremely important to be able to monitor the performance of any service. The natural inclination is to assume that the results of any research are translated into clinical practice. This is, of course, a fallacy, particularly when one considers the nature of the intervention with its many "working parts", the variability in expertise in those who interact with patients, and the need to incorporate new areas of practice. Unlike pharmacotherapy, specialist nurse-led management is not an exact science – in fact, it has a strong component of "art" as well as science.

The protocols outlined above do, as stated, attempt to provide a uniformity of high standard of care. However, it is important to audit health outcomes to ensure that a service is functioning as intended. Significantly, there is a dearth of published data to illustrate the type of audited results described below. The following audit data incorporate information from both ATHENA and a careful examination of patient outcomes according to the various sites that comprise the Glasgow service (remembering that each site was established at a different time and overall the service remains in its infancy).

Audit data

The first complete analysis of data from the Glasgow service was performed in January 2003 on the first 900 patients recruited since May 2000. Numbers varied between sites due to the service being introduced at a different time at each site over a 13-month period. Wherever possible, direct comparison of results from the Glasgow service database, with outcomes in the usual care arm of the original randomised controlled trial described in Chapters 1 and 4, were made. As described in Chapter 3, health outcomes in the usual care and intervention arms of the Glasgow trial were remarkably similar to those reported in other older and fragile patient cohorts participating in studies in the USA and Australia. As such, where results from the active intervention arm of randomised controlled trials are included within this chapter (denoted as RCT on the graphs), they are directly compared to the first 84 patients recruited into the Glasgow service on each hospital site – the same number included in the intervention arm of the study. Moreover, where appropriate, using the outcome data from the usual care arm of the study, we have indicated

Heart Failure Liaison Service
Home Visit on 18/12/2001
Ref: KR/C/

Dr Jones
Anytown Health Centre
41 Old Road
Glasgow
G36 78Z

****
****
****
****
****

Fax 0141 211 0001
Tel 0141 211 0000

Dictated: 18/12/2001
Typed: 18/12/2001

Dear Dr Jones
Re: Mrs Mary Smith, DOB 05/02/1935
101 Any Road, Glasgow

Symptoms	Signs	
NYHA Class III	BP 106/55	No ascites
No angina	Pulse 68 bpm	Ankle oedema
Progress slightly worse		

Medication	Dose	Bloods		Problems List
Isosorbide Mononitrate	60 mg mane	Na	139 mmol/l	Severe LVD
Carvedilol	6·25 mg bd	K	4·6 mmol/l	Atrial fibrillation
		Cl	101 mmol/l	Diabetes
Pravastatin Sodium	40 mg nocte	Bicarbonate	32 mmol/l	Hypercholesterolaemia
Warfarin Sodium	2 mg Sat/Sun	Urea	7·8 mmol/l	Ischaemic heart disease
Warfarin Sodium	1 mg Mon-Fri	Creatinine	100 mcmol/l	Previous VF arrest
Ramipril	5 mg nocte			
Frusemide	80 mg bd			
• Ramipril	5 mg bd			

Mrs Smith was feeling generally unwell when I visited today. Her heart failure symptoms have been unstable again recently and she has increased the diuretic dose back up to Frusemide 80mg BD. I have suggested that she try again to optimise the Ramipril dose to 5mg BD. She had previously tolerated this in terms of her renal function but stopped it due to dizziness. Her blood pressure and U&Es today are satisfactory.
I will telephone her later this week to review.

The changes to this patient's management are in accordance with the nurse liaison service medical therapy guidelines.

Yours sincerely

Return Appointment
21/12/2001
(Telephone Call)

Heart Failure Liaison Sister

CC: Medical records, GRI

Figure 6.7 Typical letter generated from ATHENA database

Table 6.2 Demographic profile of patients

	RCT	H1	H2	H3	H4	H5
Mean Age	74·4	71·8	73·9	71·5	71·8	72·5
Male	54	54	44	48	52	55
	(64%)	(64%)	(52%)	(57%)	(62%)	(65%)
Living Alone	37	37	26	31	42	26
	(44%)	(44%)	(31%)	(37%)	(50%)	(31%)

"expected" rates to compare with the actual outcomes so far determined. It is important to note that patients in the randomised study were all recruited from one hospital (H2). Other service information presented below has been gleaned from the database for the first full year's worth of data on each hospital site.

Age and sex of patients

Table 6.2 compares the age and sex of patients enrolled at each hospital in addition to the proportion who live alone and compares them to those enrolled in the original randomised trial.

Deprivation profile of patients

Based on the Carstairs Index, which scores deprivation in relation to postcode and other influencing factors such as home/car ownership and number of inhabitants per household, patients were grouped into low, medium, and high areas of deprivation. Although deprivation category was not highlighted in the randomised controlled trial, these data are an important component of demographic data collected at patient enrolment. Patients from poorer socioeconomic areas tend to have worse health outcomes and have less capacity to implement recommended changes in their lifestyle and treatment. As can be appreciated the profile of patients according to this parameter is different for each participating hospital (see Figure 6.8).

Underlying cause of heart failure

As expected, given inclusion criteria that favour those with left ventricular systolic dysfunction (predominantly men), myocardial ischaemia (69%) is currently the most commonly attributable cause of heart failure in patients within the Glasgow service. Other significant causes of heart failure include cardiomyopathies of varying underlying aetiologies (12%), hypertension (10%), and valvular dysfunction (8%).

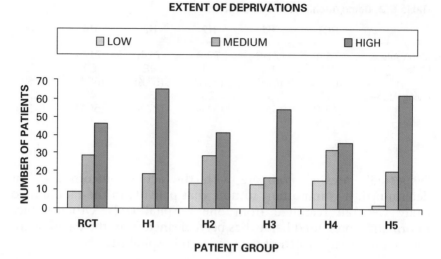

Figure 6.8 Deprivation profile of patients

All-cause, recurrent readmissions

Given that many patients recruited to the Glasgow service have a series of pre-existing comorbidities, we felt that it was important to examine the number of days they spent as a hospital inpatient during a recurrent hospital admission (after exposure to the Glasgow service) according to whether it was directly caused by heart failure or because of another condition. As can be appreciated from Figure 6.9, other conditions contribute greatly to the subsequent need for re-hospitalisation within 12 months and these also need to be addressed in the post-discharge period rather than just concentrating on chronic heart failure.

It is important to note the variable pattern of recurrent hospital stay across each service site. As expected the positive results from the original recruiting hospital (H2) are consistent with the outcomes reported in the original cohort recruited to the randomised study (the dotted line represents the expected outcome of hospital stay based on "usual care" outcomes). These positive results are replicated in H1 and H4 but not in H3 and H5 (see commentary below). Figure 6.10 shows the percentage of patients readmitted for any reason within 12 months. Clearly, in all centres, the rate of patient all-cause readmission has been reduced relative to the expected rate of 60% from the usual care cohort in the original randomised trial (once again – indicated by the dotted line).

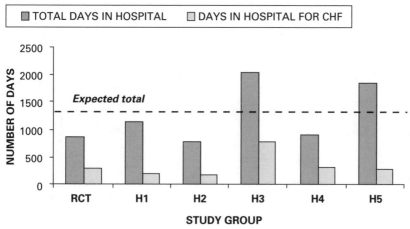

Figure 6.9 Cause of recurrent hospital stay

Figure 6.11 shows a further comparison by isolating those cases where an acute exacerbation of heart failure (for example as evidenced by acute pulmonary oedema) was clearly the principal cause of readmission within 12 months. As before, a comparison with the usual care group is indicated by the dotted line – it's important to note, however, that this an adjusted figure taking into account total readmissions rather than simply reflecting a proportion).

All-cause mortality

Ultimately, improved survival and quality of life are major objectives of the Glasgow service. A preliminary analysis of one-year all-cause mortality data is presented in Figure 6.12. Across the city, every one of the five hospitals recorded greater survival than was demonstrated by the randomised study (both cohorts) thus providing valuable evidence that the provision of specialist nurses is indeed a most effective way of caring for patients in the community with chronic heart failure.

Service activity

Patient contact is the most important component of the Glasgow service and, in order to monitor the amount of contacts occurring, in the audit we divided them into various contact types – an important caveat is that not all sites operate nurse-led clinics. The data presented in Figure 6.13 refer to the first full year of operation for each hospital

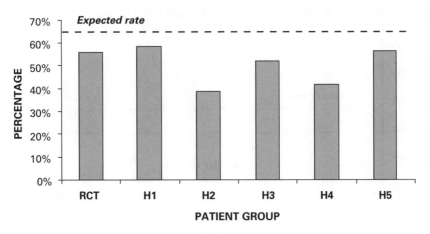

Figure 6.10   Rate of all-cause readmission within 12 months

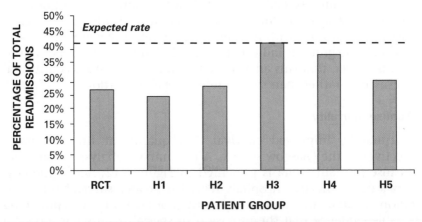

Figure 6.11   Readmissions caused by worsening heart failure

and show the various types of patient contact undertaken. As expected, home visits represent the major component of service activity.

Obviously, pharmacology plays a huge part in the effectiveness of the service provided and the range of initiation and titration issues that need to be addressed in order to ensure that patients are receiving gold standard pharmacotherapy can greatly add to the overall workload of the service. Figure 6.14 highlights the overall number of

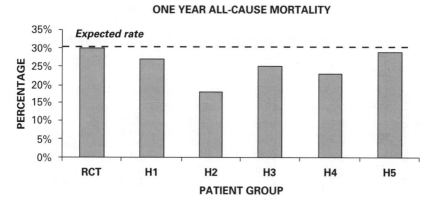

Figure 6.12 One year all-cause mortality rates

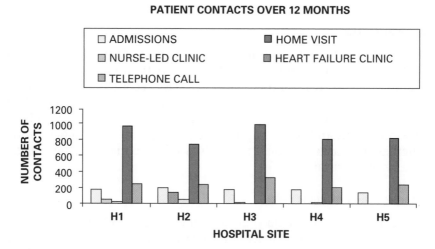

Figure 6.13 Number and types of patient contact

interventions prescribed by the heart failure nurses in year 1 of their service for all drug therapies.

Not surprisingly, loop diuretics and angiotensin converting enzyme inhibitors were responsible for the majority of the interventions. However, it is important to note that these data were largely collected before the widespread initiation of β-blockers – a class of agents that requires careful titration. Moreover, the addition of angiotensin receptor blockers to the armoury of agents used to treat chronic heart failure (see Chapter 2) is likely to increase such activity.

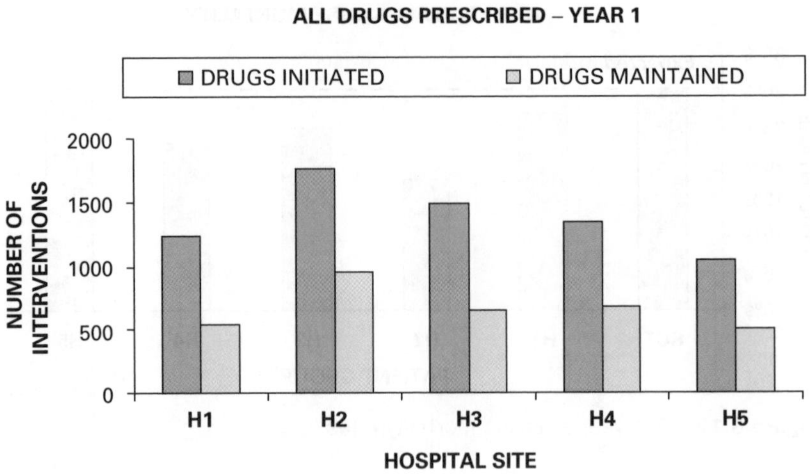

ALL DRUGS PRESCRIBED – YEAR 1

Figure 6.14 Overall drug interventions

Clinical status

In addition to outcome and service activity data, the audit also captures individual parameters relating to patient clinical status. For example, Figure 6.15 shows "current" (last recorded measurement) levels of left ventricular systolic impairment in patients exposed to the Glasgow service. Clearly, there is potential to monitor trends in relation to this and other important clinical parameters to determine whether the service is able to alter, in a positive manner, the natural history of heart failure.

Interpretation of audit data

Overall, these audit data provide useful insights (warts and all) into the overall activity and impact of the Glasgow service. Compared to the reported rates of activity in the active intervention and usual care cohort arms of the randomised study, most sites are performing extremely well. This is particularly so given the fact that they appear to be recruiting more patients from lower socioeconomic areas and with greater levels of comorbidity likely to increase the probability of morbidity and mortality. If anything, it highlights, once again, the value of designing and applying interventions that can meet the flexible needs of a local population and the healthcare services provided to them.

As stated before, translating research into practice (particularly on a large scale) is extremely difficult. The site with the worst health outcomes overall, as measured by the number of patients admitted for recurrent heart failure, highlights the value of auditing a service. Since it was discovered that less than optimal outcomes were occurring the

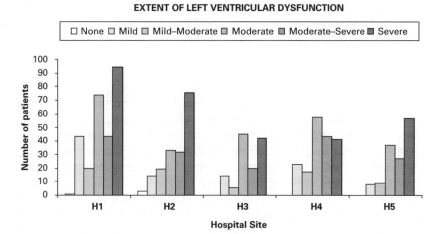

EXTENT OF LEFT VENTRICULAR DYSFUNCTION

□ None □ Mild □ Mild–Moderate □ Moderate ■ Moderate–Severe ■ Severe

Figure 6.15 Extent of left ventricular systolic dysfunction.

service provided there was re-evaluated and a number of changes implemented. Significantly, recent audit data have demonstrated improved health outcomes relative to the data shown above.

In order to monitor activity across the five sites of the Glasgow service we have now instituted a quarterly audit programme. Data are collated from each site using specific queries written into the ATHENA program that mirror the type of data presented in the graphs above.

The difference between clinical audit and clinical effectiveness: a focus on quality of life

Whilst clinical audit enables us to monitor and measure service workloads and interventions it also facilitates a review of the clinical effectiveness of the Glasgow service using high quality, hard outcome data (for example morbidity and mortality related outcomes) to:

- improve practice
- undertake research
- identify particularly effective components of intervention
- facilitate changes in clinical practice
- identify clinical gaps in the service and respond accordingly.

As stated, promoting a patient-focused service is a key priority and it was noted that patient quality of life was a time-consuming but important parameter to measure in terms of monitoring the effectiveness of the Glasgow service. A heart failure specific quality of life measurement tool is currently being piloted in the service (the LVD-36 – Figure 6.16) in order to provide such data.

Summary

Establishing the Glasgow Heart Failure Liaison Service entailed a substantial amount of time and effort – all well spent. The protocols outlined in this and other chapters are designed to match patient intervention and health outcomes with the stated intentions of the service, irrespective of where and by whom it is being delivered.

Now that we are auditing the service regularly it is becoming clear where potential problem areas could lie. Had we had a clear discharge policy from the beginning some of our current problems with large, labour intensive caseloads may not have arisen. However in identifying the pitfalls and gaps in our service we are developing a safe and structured discharge policy for stable patients with an open pathway of referral back into the service if required.

If new developments (for example expanding the patient base to those with so-called diastolic heart failure) were to result in additional new referrals it would become even more necessary to follow guidelines strictly and to discharge patients when appropriate to allow for expansion of the service. Moreover, it is important to know that the service is able to incorporate new treatment options (ranging from newer pharmacological agents in heart failure such as the angiotensin receptor blockers to modes of management including "palliative care") without compromising the overall cost-effectiveness of the service.

Thus far, the audit data (both those presented and newer data demonstrating positive directions for all important outcomes) show that the Glasgow service is providing a quality healthcare service.

*Please answer the following questions as you are feeling **these days**. Tick either true or false for each question.*

Because of my heart condition:	True	False
I suffer with tired legs	☐	☐
I suffer with nausea (feeling sick)	☐	☐
I suffer with swollen legs	☐	☐

Because of my heart condition:	True	False
I am afraid that if I go out I will be short of breath	☐	☐
I am frightened to do too much in case I become short of breath	☐	☐
I get out of breath with the least physical exercise	☐	☐
I am frightened to push myself too far	☐	☐
I take a long time to get washed or dressed	☐	☐

If you do not do these activities for any reason other than your heart condition, then please tick false

Because of my heart condition:	True	False
I have difficulty running, such as for a bus	☐	☐
I have difficulty either jogging, exercising or dancing	☐	☐
I have difficulty playing with children/grandchildren	☐	☐
I have difficulty either mowing the lawn or hoovering/vacuum cleaning	☐	☐

Because of my heart condition:	True	False
I feel exhausted	☐	☐
I feel low in energy	☐	☐
I feel sleepy or drowsy	☐	☐
I need to rest more	☐	☐
I feel that everything is an effort	☐	☐
My muscles feel weak	☐	☐
I get cold easily	☐	☐
I wake up frequently during the night	☐	☐
I have become frail or an invalid	☐	☐

Because of my heart condition:	True	False
I feel frustrated	☐	☐
I feel nervous	☐	☐
I feel irritable	☐	☐
I feel restless	☐	☐
I feel out of control of my life	☐	☐
I feel that I can not enjoy a full life	☐	☐
I've lost confidence in myself	☐	☐

Because of my heart condition:	True	False
I have difficulty having a regular social life	☐	☐
There are places I would like to go to but can't	☐	☐
I worry that going on holiday could make my heart condition worse	☐	☐
I have had to alter my lifestyle	☐	☐
I am restricted in fulfilling my family duties	☐	☐
I feel dependent on others	☐	☐

	True	False
I find it a real nuisance having to take tablets for my heart condition	☐	☐
My heart condition stops me doing things that I would like to do	☐	☐

PLEASE CHECK THAT YOU HAVE ANSWERED ALL THE QUESTIONS
THANK YOU FOR YOUR TIME

Figure 6.16   LVD-36

7: Assessing the patient with heart failure

MARGARET B MCENTEGART, ERIC GRAY

Introduction

As described in more detail in Chapter 1, chronic heart failure is a major cause of morbidity and mortality in westernised society and is rapidly becoming a global epidemic.[1] The increasing prevalence of heart failure is largely attributable to the ageing population and improved survival post myocardial infarction.[2] Heart failure is associated with high rates of hospital readmission and, largely because of this, has become a major burden on healthcare resources, accounting for 1–2% of healthcare expenditure in the UK.[3] Recognition of this exponentially rising demand has lead to the development of new approaches to the management of heart failure. The emergence of the role of the heart failure specialist nurse is a valuable addition to existing medical services providing cost-effective and improved care for the patient with heart failure (see Chapters 3 and 5 for more details). In providing rapid assessment and response to changes in patients' heart failure status, hospital readmission rates and inpatient days are reduced and the patients can be managed in their home environment.

Assessing a patient with heart failure involves the same principles as assessing any other patient: those of history taking, clinical examination, and performing appropriate investigations. The formal clinical assessment of patients has traditionally been undertaken by doctors, following a systematic approach (i.e. cardiovascular, respiratory, abdominal, and neurological systems), while nursing assessment has traditionally been based on a more comprehensive history, the monitoring of objective observations, and a more gradual gathering of first-hand information. With the increasing role of the specialist nurse throughout health care, a marrying of these two approaches is required. Many of these roles are disease specific (for example heart failure, fast-track chest pain and chronic obstructive pulmonary disease nurse specialists) with the aim, therefore, of employing a disease specific approach to the assessment, while drawing on experience to place this in the context of the patient's general health. Heart failure usually manifests itself as a combination of well described symptoms and signs lending itself to this type of approach.

The diagnosis and assessment of heart failure

Heart failure is a clinical diagnosis made on the basis of the history, examination, and appropriate investigations. The European Society of Cardiology task force stated that the diagnosis of heart failure requires the presence of typical symptoms and objective evidence of cardiac dysfunction at rest.[4] Once the diagnosis is established ongoing assessment of the patient with heart failure involves the same clinical skills.

History taking

In obtaining a history the presenting complaint, history of presenting complaint, past medical history, drug history, family history, and social history should be sought. The presenting complaint describes the patient's currently troublesome symptoms. In addition to a detailed account of the development and nature of these, symptoms of heart failure should be specifically sought. The key symptoms of heart failure are listed below.

Key symptoms of heart failure

Dyspnoea
Orthopnoea
Paroxysmal nocturnal dyspnoea
Lethargy/fatigue
Ankle swelling

Abdominal swelling
Anorexia
Nocturnal cough
Wheeze

Presenting complaint

Exertional breathlessness and fatigue are the two most commonly reported symptoms in heart failure, and together lead to exercise intolerance. Breathlessness (dyspnoea) is the most sensitive symptom in diagnosing heart failure (i.e. If the patient is not breathless he or she is unlikely to have heart failure). The grading of its severity using the New York Heart Asssociation (NYHA) classification (see below) is the most prognostically important factor in the clinical history.

New York Heart Association (NYHA) classification of heart failure

Class I
No limitation during ordinary activity

Class II
Slight limitation during ordinary activity

Class III
Marked limitation of normal activities without symptoms at rest

Class IV
Unable to undertake physical activity without symptoms. Symptoms at rest

In decompensated heart failure, breathlessness is largely attributed to pulmonary oedema due to increased pulmonary capillary pressures. On lying down the pulmonary venous pressure increases further and causes orthopnoea. This may progress to acute nocturnal attacks of breathlessness waking the patient from sleep (paroxysmal nocturnal dyspnoea). Despite normal fluid balance (euvolaemia) patients with chronic heart failure may still feel breathless. The cause of this is not fully understood, but is thought to be related to reduced tissue perfusion, abnormal function of the cardiopulmonary receptors, and to respiratory muscle fatigue.

When assessing breathlessness it is important to consider any possible contributing comorbidities (for example asthma/chronic obstructive pulmonary disease) and to determine the "normal" baseline for that particular individual. The aim of the assessment is to determine whether there has been any deterioration from this baseline or whether there has been a positive response to therapy

Fatigue in chronic heart failure is thought to be attributable to reduced cardiac reserve on exercise, inadequate perfusion of exercising muscles, and abnormal skeletal muscle function.[5]

Ankle swelling is the next most commonly reported symptom, and the other defining symptom of heart failure. Patients may also report active symptoms related to the aetiology of their heart failure (for example decubitus angina or angina pectoris) or to co-existing cardiac or respiratory problems (for example palpitations, cough, and wheeze).

Past medical history

A past medical history, particularly any prior history of cardiac disease, the presence of cardiovascular risk factors, or important comorbidities, should be obtained.

Past medical history

Angina
Myocardial infarction
Coronary angiography
Coronary artery bypass graft
Arrhythmia
Valvular disease

Risk factors

Hypertension
Hypercholesterolaemia
Diabetes mellitus
Smoking
Alcohol excess

Comorbidities

Cerebrovascular disease
Peripheral vascular disease
Chronic renal failure
Chronic obstructive pulmonary disease/asthma

Drug history A detailed drug history should be documented. This should be reviewed to identify sub-optimal heart failure therapy and/or inappropriate therapy. This may include the absence or sub-optimal doses of ACE inhibitor, angiotensin receptor blocker, or β-blocker therapy. The appropriateness of spironolactone and digoxin therapy as adjunctive therapy and the inappropriate prescription of non-steroidal anti-inflammatory drugs should be assessed. The use of drug therapy which acts to lower the blood pressure and is of no benefit in the management of heart failure should be reviewed as these may need to be discontinued to allow optimisation of ACE inhibitor, angiotensin receptor blocker, and β-blocker therapy.

Family history The presence of a family history of premature cardiac disease or any other conditions should be sought. This may, in some cases, be the only concrete reason to suspect the development of heart failure in the absence of more definitive investigations.

Social history The details of a patient's social circumstances are of particular importance when managing chronic disease in the home environment. Assessing the patient in that environment allows a more representative assessment of heart failure status and of the need for further support. These issues will be addressed elsewhere in this book.

Examination

The clinical examination of the patient with heart failure, as performed by a heart failure specialist nurse in the community, currently involves assessment of the patient's general condition, degree of breathlessness and fatigue, and examination of the pulse, blood pressure, presence or absence of oedema, and monitoring of their weight. With the potential in the future for this to be extended into a more comprehensive, disease specific assessment of heart failure status, that is what we will describe here.

Key clinical signs of heart failure

Tachycardia
Pulsus alternans
Hypotension
Elevated jugular venous pressure
Displaced apex beat
Third heart sound
Dyspnoea/tachypnoea
Crepitations
Wheeze
Oedema
Hepatomegaly
Ascites
Cachexia and muscle wasting

The first observation made when examining any patient is an impression of their general condition. On first meeting a patient this is important to allow you to place their disease in context and to define a baseline of their condition. Thereafter, at further assessments, knowing the patient from previous meetings, an overall impression can be obtained of whether they have improved, appear stable, or have deteriorated.

Pulse and blood pressure

The pulse and blood pressure are markers of a patient's haemodynamic stability. When examining the pulse the radial artery is used, unless absent bilaterally, when a more proximal artery, typically the brachial or carotid, can be assessed. The blood pressure is usually measured in the upper arm, using the brachial artery, with the patient either sitting or lying. Lying and standing blood pressure should be performed in a patient reporting symptoms suggestive of postural hypotension. A fall in systolic blood pressure of >20 mmHg on standing is significant.

Pulse

The rate and rhythm are of particular interest and should be documented.

Rate The normal heart rate is defined as 60–100 bpm, with bradycardia defined as < 60 bpm, and tachycardia as >100 bpm. Tachycardia is part of the heart's normal response to increased sympathetic activity and therefore can be induced physiologically for example by anxiety, fear, or pain. In the patient with heart failure the heart rate tends to rise with the compensatory activation of the sympathetic nervous system. In mild or moderate heart failure the patient is unlikely to be tachycardic. This may develop in severe heart failure but may be absent particularly in the presence of β-blocker therapy. Tachycardia can also be a relatively late sign of decompensating heart failure and other signs of this should be sought.

Bradycardia in a patient with heart failure is most commonly due to β-blocker therapy. This is a desired effect reflecting inhibition of sympathetic activity. It may in some patients prohibit maximisation of β-blocker therapy to the target doses recommended in clinical trials. The presence of bradycardia in the absence of β-blocker therapy prohibits their use and needs further investigation initially with a 12-lead ECG. In this predominantly elderly population, sick sinus syndrome and heart block should be excluded as possible underlying causes.

Rhythm Atrial fibrillation is the most common arrhythmia seen in patients with heart failure. Instead of the sino-atrial node initiating ordered electrical depolarisation this process is chaotic, resulting in irregular electrical conduction through the atrio-ventricular node and irregular ventricular depolarisation and contraction, generating an irregular pulse. The pulse is often described as "irregularly irregular", meaning there is no pattern to the irregularity and that the pulse is irregular in both rhythm and volume (see Figure 7.1). A patient with atrial fibrillation may be asymptomatic or may report palpitations, or more non-specifically breathlessness or fatigue. Palpitations are most commonly described as an awareness of the heart racing or beating irregularly or as a sensation of fluttering or thumping in the chest.

Ectopic beats (both atrial and ventricular) are common in heart failure. The patient will have a regular pulse with occasional early beats followed by a short pause before the pulse returns to being regular. Ectopics can occur regularly, after every normal beat (bigeminy) or after every two normal beats (trigeminy). In these cases the pulse feels "regularly irregular" in that there is a pattern to the irregularity (see Figure 7.2). Ectopics are usually described by patients as "missed" or "dropped beats" or as a brief pause in their heart beat followed by a pronounced thump or "jump start".

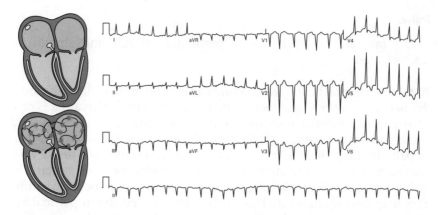

Figure 7.1 Electrical conduction in sinus rhythm and atrial fibrillation. ECG of atrial fibrillation

If the pulse is noted to be irregular a prior established history of an arrhythmia should be sought and if no history is documented an ECG performed to further define the cause.

Volume/character The volume and character of the pulse can also be described. In severe heart failure the pulse may alternate from being strong and bounding to weak and thready. This is known as *pulsus alternans* and is due to changes in the stroke volume. These beat to beat variations in stroke volume reflect changes in cardiac contractility and alteration in ventricular preload.

Blood pressure

Blood pressure monitoring plays a central role in the management of heart failure. The presence of hypotension or hypertension is important. The blood pressure in a patient with heart failure will be influenced by a number of factors including the degree of left ventricular systolic dysfunction, a prior history of hypertension, and the anti-hypertensive effects of drug therapy.

In the early stages of heart failure left ventricular systolic function is usually adequate to generate a cardiac output sufficient to sustain arterial pressure, and the blood pressure most commonly is normal. As heart failure progresses and the cardiac output decreases compensatory activation of the renin–angiotensin–aldosterone system and sympathetic nervous system work to sustain an adequate circulating volume and blood pressure. As heart failure progresses further these auto-regulatory mechanisms become detrimental to the heart's attempts to maintain haemodynamic stability, and hypotension develops. Inhibition of these autoregulatory mechanisms (with ACE

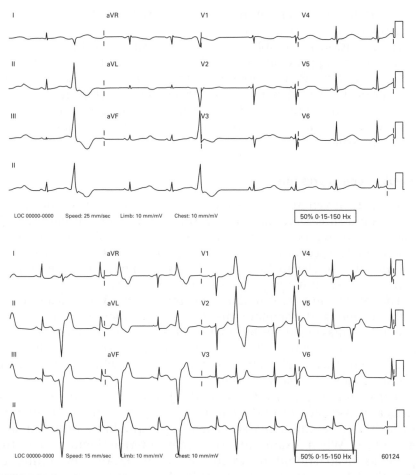

Figure 7.2 ECGs showing sinus rhythm with ventricular ectopics and ventricular bigeminy

inhibitors, angiotensin receptor blockers (ARB) and β-blockers) is therefore important before this point of physiological decompensation is reached.

Systolic hypotension is defined as systolic blood pressure < 100 mmHg. Hypotension may result in hypoperfusion of the organs resulting, for example, in the brain to collapse or lightheadedness, or in the kidneys to deterioration in renal function. ACE inhibitors, ARBs, β-blockers, and diuretics all lower the blood pressure and in some patients hypotension prohibits their use or optimisation. The commencement of these drugs in the early stages of heart failure is important to ensure they are haemodynamically tolerated. Due to the recognised mortality benefits from optimised therapy, systolic blood pressure lower than usually considered adequate may be acceptable in the heart failure patient in the absence of any associated symptoms or deterioration in renal function.

Hypertension is variably defined with a sustained blood pressure >140/85 mmHg generally accepted in clinical practice. Hypertensive cardiomyopathy is an important cause of heart failure, but once significant left ventricular systolic dysfunction develops it is unusual for the hypertension to persist. In addition, as discussed above, heart failure therapy has the dual benefit in these patients of lowering the blood pressure.

Jugular venous pressure

The jugular venous pressure (JVP) is a clinical measure of the central venous pressure. Determination of the JVP is a difficult clinical skill and while its reproducibility is high amongst cardiologists it is much lower in non-specialists. It has a good positive predictive value (i.e. if it is noted to be elevated the patient is likely to have heart failure) but is not elevated in many patients with heart failure.

The internal jugular vein drains via the superior vena cava into the right atrium and therefore the degree to which it is filled and distended, making it visible in the neck, is a marker of the right atrial/central pressure. If a patient with heart failure is fluid overloaded their right atrial/central pressure will become raised leading to a visibly elevated JVP.

It is common practice to assess the JVP on the right side of the neck as valves present in the left internal jugular vein are thought to make it a less accurate marker. The patient should be sitting up at a 45° angle. When examining the right internal jugular vein the patient's head should be tilted slightly backward and round to face the left (i.e. away from the side of the neck being examined). The internal jugular vein runs up between the two heads of the sternocleidomastoid muscle towards the angle of the jaw and the earlobe (see Figure 7.3).

There are a number of ways to help determine that the vessel identified is indeed the internal jugular vein and not for example the external jugular vein or carotid artery. Firstly, if the vessel is venous you should be able to compress and obliterate it and it should not have a palpable pulse. Secondly, if the vessel is emptied by milking it upwards towards the angle of the jaw and then released, with it being venous, it will fill from above draining towards the heart. If doubt remains, further confirmation can be sought by performing the hepatojugular reflex. This test involves exerting firm but gentle pressure over the right subcostal area while observing the JVP. This action increases pressure in the liver, which increases venous return from the liver to the right atrium, which subsequently causes the JVP to visibly rise further. Patients with heart failure may have a degree of

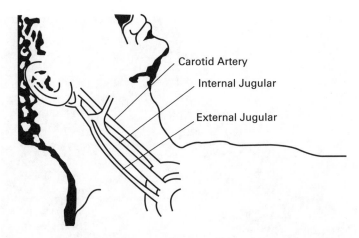

Carotid Artery

Internal Jugular

External Jugular

Figure 7.3 Anatomy of the major neck vessels

liver congestion and it is important to avoid precipitating discomfort when performing this test (see Figure 7.4).

Praecordium

The anterior chest wall should be inspected for scars indicating previous cardiac surgery (for example coronary artery bypass grafts or valve replacement). Gynaecomastia (enlargement of the breasts) is a recognised reversible side effect of spironolactone in males. Patients will often report the associated breast discomfort when this clinical sign should be specifically looked for.

Apex beat

The apex beat is the point of maximum palpable pulsation on the praecordium. This should be at the fifth intercostal space in the midclavicular line. It is located by placing the fingers of a flat palm in the midaxillary line centred over the fifth intercostal space and slowly moving round towards the midclavicular line until the pulsation is located. In some patients with thick chest walls the apex is impalpable. In heart failure the heart can become dilated and with this the apex is displaced downwards and outwards into the axilla. The nature of the apex beat can also be described. In heart failure it may be felt to be diffuse, rather than well localised, or to be particularly forceful.

Heart sounds

In auscultation of the normal heart there are two heart sounds, S_1 and S_2. S_1 is produced by closure of the mitral and tricuspid valves,

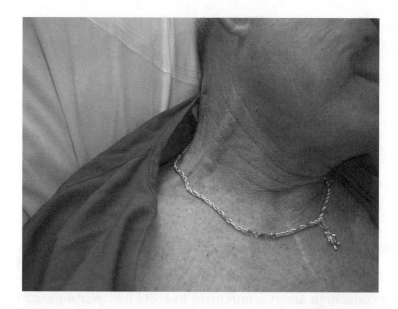

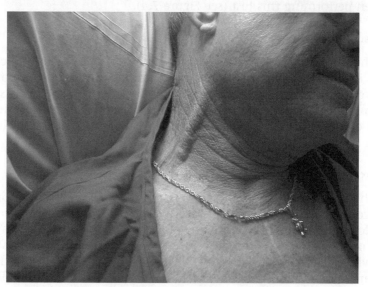

Figure 7.4 The JVP and the hepatojugular reflex

and S_2 by closure of the aortic and pulmonary valves. In a patient with heart failure auscultation is important to identify the presence of a third heart sound and any murmurs signifying possible valvular disease. A third heart sound (S_3) may be caused in decompensated heart failure by rapid ventricular filling and together with a tachycardia produces a "gallop" rhythm (this is classically described as sounding like a horse galloping).

Valvular disease is important both as a cause and as a consequence of heart failure. Mitral regurgitation and aortic stenosis can both eventually lead to the development of cardiomyopathy which may be prevented if valve replacement or repair is undertaken at the appropriate time. Patients with heart failure of other aetiologies, associated with left ventricular dilation, a regional wall motion abnormality, or a papillary muscle rupture can develop functional mitral regurgitation. In functional mitral regurgitation the valve itself is normal but the coaptation of the leaflets is abnormal due to changes in the structure of the ventricle or annulus. The resultant mitral regurgitation can improve with improvement of left ventricular dimensions and function.

Both mitral regurgitation and aortic stenosis are systolic murmurs heard between S_1 and S_2. Mitral regurgitation is described as a "pansystolic" murmur in that it is heard throughout systole, sometimes obscuring the heart sounds, and is constant in intensity. Aortic stenosis is described as an "ejection systolic" murmur in that it begins immediately after S_1, builds up in intensity to mid systole, and stops sharply allowing S_2 to be heard. If on auscultation a murmur is suspected any known history of valvular disease should be sought and the most recent echocardiography report reviewed. If the murmur appears to be new an updated echocardiogram should be performed.

Respiration and breath sounds

In assessing a patient's respiration the first thing to note is whether they appear breathless at rest or on exertion. Inability to complete sentences due to breathlessness can be elicited by specifically asking open-ended questions. The respiratory rate should be recorded to establish whether it is increased (tachypnoea being a respiratory rate > 14 breaths per minute).

Examination of the lungs is most commonly performed from the back of the chest. For a complete respiratory examination the front of the chest should also be examined but in the heart failure assessment, where we are particularly interested in the lung bases, examination from the back is adequate. The posterior chest wall should be inspected for scars and for symmetry of chest wall movement with respiration. Percussion and auscultation should be performed throughout both lung fields comparing one side with the other and listening round into the axillae where the lung bases are best heard.

Percussion over normal air-filled lung fields produces a resonant sound. A collection of fluid between the chest wall and lung (i.e. a pleural effusion), or an area of consolidation (most commonly due to infection) will be dull to percussion. In decompensated heart failure fluid may accumulate in the chest in the form of a pleural effusion. Due to gravitational force effusions will form initially at the lung bases.

On auscultation air entry throughout both lung fields and the presence of any abnormal respiratory sounds should be assessed. It is important to ask the patient to take deep breaths through the mouth to avoid misinterpretation of shallow respiration. Air entry will be reduced where there is a pleural effusion, an area of consolidation, or lobar collapse, as sound is not transmitted through fluid or solid. If a pleural effusion is suspected from percussion and auscultation this can be further assessed by performing vocal resonance. This involves auscultating the lung fields while the patient quietly says "99". This sound normally resonates through the lungs and is clearly heard on auscultation but, as with the breath sounds, will not be heard over an effusion.

The most common abnormal respiratory sounds in heart failure are crepitations (also known as crackles or rales). Crepitations are caused by fluid in the lung air spaces (alveoli). These are usually initially heard at the lung bases and progress up through the lung fields as pulmonary oedema progresses. When crepitations are heard the patient should be asked to cough before listening again to ensure the added sounds were not due to secretions in the upper airways, as these can produce a similar sound. Crepitations have a low positive predictive value (i.e. their detection does not necessarily indicate the presence of heart failure) and high inter-observer difference in detection.

Oedema

Fluid retention in heart failure is initiated by the fall in cardiac output leading to activation of the sodium-retaining renin–angiotensin-aldosterone and sympathetic nervous systems. Increased pressure in the venous system is distributed retrogradely to the smaller vessels, precipitating transudation of fluid into the soft tissues and producing bilateral oedema that is pitting in nature. It is estimated that oedema is usually clinically detectable once approximately 5 litres of excess fluid volume has accumulated, which translates approximately to a weight gain of 5 kg. It is important when examining for oedema that visual assessment alone is not relied upon. Gentle pressure should be exerted on any affected areas for 2 or 3 seconds and if pitting oedema is present the pressure marks persist after pressure is withdrawn. Due to gravitational force the ankles are usually the first site where oedema is detected, spreading proximally as fluid accumulates (see Figure 7.5). It can also occur in the sacral area, scrotum, abdominal wall, periorbitally, and in the upper limbs. In a patient who is bed bound

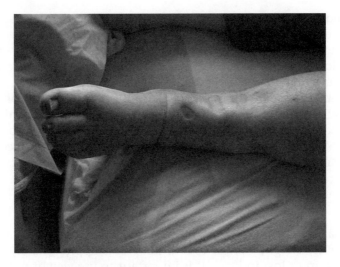

Figure 7.5   Lower limb pitting oedema

sacral oedema should be specifically looked for even in the absence
of lower limb oedema.

Ascites

Fluid can also accumulate in the abdominal cavity as ascites. The
development of ascites is insidious with slowly increasing abdominal
girth, which may be noticed as a progressive increase in belt size or with
clothes becoming too tight. On standing the fluid settles in the lower
abdomen, when lying supine the fluid can sometimes be seen to bulge
in the flanks, and when lying on one side the fluid settles in the
dependent lower side of the abdominal cavity. This is a more
pronounced feature of right heart failure but is also seen when the
primary problem is left ventricular failure. Several litres of fluid need to
be present in the abdominal cavity before it is clinically detectable. The
presence of ascites can be confirmed by eliciting the sign of shifting
dullness. With the examiner standing on the right side of the supine
patient the abdomen is percussed repeatedly from the umbilicus out
towards the left flank (i.e. away from the examiner). Gas filled bowel
floats on top of the ascitic fluid and is resonant. The point at which the
percussion note becomes dull is marked with a pen. The patient is then
rolled on their right side towards the examiner. After 30 seconds or so in
this position, allowing time for fluid shift, the percussion is repeated
finding that the area that was previously dull has become resonant as

any fluid in the left flank has now shifted to the right flank. This is shifting dullness and confirms the presence of ascites.

Increased venous pressures in heart failure can result in liver congestion. This can progress to cause liver enlargement (hepatomegaly) and derangement of liver function tests. The liver is usually impalpable, not extending below the right costal margin of the rib cage. When it enlarges significantly it becomes palpable and can be described by how many centimetres it extends below the costal margin. When hepatomegaly is due to congestion the surface of the liver is smooth, it is dull to percussion, and it may be tender.

Weight

Regular weight monitoring is established as a method of assessing fluid status. Weight gain or loss in kilograms approximately equates to fluid gain or loss in litres. It is important to use weight monitoring in conjunction with symptoms and other signs found on examination as sometimes weight change may be due to change in the patient's dry weight. Follow-up with daily weight and symptom monitoring using a technology based system has been shown to reduce mortality in advanced heart failure.[6]

In severe chronic heart failure, as in other chronic diseases (for example chronic obstructive pulmonary disease, chronic renal failure), some patients develop marked weight loss. This process is known as cardiac cachexia. Cachectic heart failure patients have the greatest symptomatic limitation and a very poor prognosis with mortality rates of 50% at 18 months.[7] The pathophysiological mechanisms involved in this systemic wasting process remain unclear.

Other considerations

In diagnosing heart failure none of the symptoms or signs in isolation is sensitive or specific but the assessment becomes so when they are taken in combination and may allow a clinical diagnosis to be made with some confidence (see Table 7.1).[8]

There are a number of conditions that will present with some of the symptoms or signs of heart failure and if assessment is incomplete may be misdiagnosed as heart failure. Anaemia will cause fatigue and breathlessness. If a patient becomes profoundly anaemic a hyperdynamic state can be induced, as can also occur in hyperthyroidism. Alternatively, hypothyroidism can cause fatigue and oedema, as can any cause of sodium and water retention (for example renal failure, liver failure, or drugs).

Making an accurate diagnosis of heart failure is known to be particularly difficult in women, the obese, and the elderly. Obesity

Table 7.1 Sensitivity and specificity of symptoms and signs for diagnosing heart failure

Symptom or sign	Sensitivity (%)	Specificity (%)	Predictive accuracy (%)
Exertional dyspnoea	66	52	23
Orthopnoea	21	81	2
Paroxysmal nocturnal dyspnoea	33	76	26
History of oedema	23	80	22
Resting heart rate > 100 bpm	7	99	6
Rales	13	91	21
Third heart sound	31	95	61
Jugular venous distension	10	97	2
Oedema (on examination)	10	93	3

may be associated with symptoms of breathlessness, fatigue, and ankle swelling in the context of sub-optimal clinical examination and investigations. The presence of multiple comorbidities in the elderly (for example chronic obstructive pulmonary disease, chronic venous insufficiency) can complicate the clinical picture and interpretation of investigations.

Therefore, in order to firmly establish the diagnosis it is essential to obtain a detailed history, perform a comprehensive examination and proceed to the appropriate investigations.

Investigations

Chest radiograph

The chest radiograph, in detecting the presence of cardiomegaly and pulmonary venous congestion, has a high predictive value for heart failure when taken together with the clinical assessment and the ECG. Cardiomegaly is defined as a cardiothoracic ratio of >0·50. Signs of pulmonary congestion include upper lobe venous diversion, and interstitial and alveolar oedema (see Figure 7.6). There is known to be inter-observer variation in chest x ray film interpretation. If heart failure is suspected from the symptoms and signs but the chest x ray film and ECG are normal it is unlikely to be the diagnosis.

Electrocardiography

The ECG may reveal evidence of ischaemic heart disease (in particular a previous myocardial infarction), left ventricular hypertrophy or an

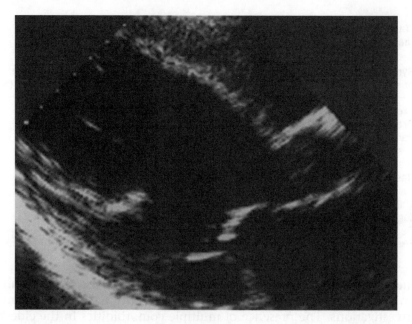

Figure 7.6 Chest radiograph showing cardiomegaly and pulmonary oedema

associated arrhythmia (most commonly atrial fibrillation). A normal ECG is rare in a patient with heart failure with left ventricular systolic dysfunction with a negative predictive value of >90%. Even in the absence of heart failure an abnormal ECG should precipitate echocardiography to assess left ventricular and valvular function.

Echocardiography

The next step is to determine cardiac function and echocardiography is the preferred and most widely used method (see Figure 7.7). Once cardiac dysfunction is confirmed echocardiography can help further in the characterisation of the heart failure and in determining the aetiology. This is important to guide management and further investigations.

The diagnosis of heart failure with left ventricular systolic dysfunction

Unless specified as isolated right heart failure, the term heart failure has essentially become synonymous with heart failure due to left ventricular dysfunction. Left ventricular dysfunction can be systolic or diastolic and this can be determined in most patients by echocardiography. Data from epidemiological studies and clinical trials show that approximately 50% of heart failure with left ventricular dysfunction is due to left ventricular systolic dysfunction with the other 50% of

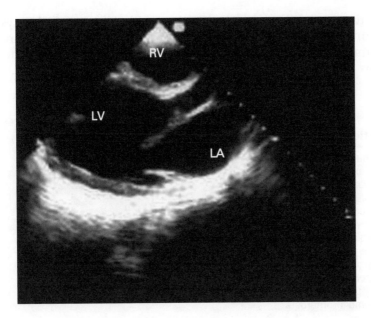

Figure 7.7 Two-dimensional echocardiogram of dilated left ventricle in patient with heart failure

patients having heart failure with preserved left ventricular systolic function (so called diastolic dysfunction). This distinction is important as the large body of evidence for heart failure therapy (as described in Chapter 2) is largely specific to the population with heart failure with left ventricular systolic dysfunction. It is also important to note that the evidence in support of nurse-led initiatives in heart failure has largely (but not exclusively) focused on those with some form of evidence of systolic impairment. Thus, there is a significant gap in the evidence regarding the management of a considerable population of patients with heart failure. With this having been recognised clinical trials are under way. Indeed, the outcome of the first large clinical trial looking at the role of angiotensin receptor blocker therapy in heart failure with preserved left ventricular systolic function (CHARM-Preserved) has been reported very recently and is discussed elsewhere in this book.

The left ventricular ejection fraction is the most frequently used measure of left ventricular systolic function. It can be assessed on echocardiogram in a number of ways (most commonly by M-mode or the modified Simpson's biplane method) but reproducibility is known to be poor. Visual grading of left ventricular systolic dysfunction into mild, moderate, and severe is widely used but is entirely subjective and difficult to standardise.

With the diagnosis of heart failure with left ventricular systolic dysfunction established the echocardiogram can also provide information regarding the aetiology of the heart failure. The box below lists the most common causes of heart failure in the UK.

Aetiology of heart failure

Ischaemic heart disease
Hypertensive heart disease
Valvular heart disease
Viral cardiomyopathy
Idiopathic cardiomyopathy
Tachyarrhythmia/bradyarrhythmia
Cardiac depressant drugs
Anaemia
Thyrotoxicosis
Hypertrophic cardiomyopathy
Postpartum cardiomyopathy
Haemochromatosis

An abnormality of the left ventricular regional wall motion would suggest ischaemia with a previous myocardial infarction in that territory, while a globally dilated left ventricle with no specific wall motion abnormality would point to a dilated cardiomyopathy. The presence of left ventricular hypertrophy may suggest prior hypertension, and the detection of significant mitral or aortic disease may suggest a valvular aetiology. In addition, the echocardiogram can provide information regarding atrial size, estimated pulmonary artery pressure, presence of mural thrombus, and the pericardium.

Haematology and biochemistry

Haematology and biochemistry blood tests should be performed as part of the diagnostic and follow-up assessment. A full blood count is important to exclude anaemia. Recent data from Glasgow have shown that anaemia is significantly more common in hospitalised heart failure patients than in the general hospitalised patient population.

Baseline renal function is important to exclude renal failure as the cause of fluid overload or as an important comorbidity, as is frequently the case in patients with diabetes or widespread vascular disease. Renal dysfunction secondary to heart failure is common and due to reduced renal perfusion and/or the nephrotoxic effects of the treatment. The urea, creatinine, and electrolytes should be regularly monitored.

The liver function tests should be checked to exclude hepatic congestion. Thyroid function tests are important to exclude both hyperthyroidism and hypothyroidism. Viral serology and ferritin should be checked as part of aetiology screening.

Natriuretic peptide

Of the natriuretic peptides studied B-type natriuretic peptide (BNP) has emerged as the most useful diagnostic and prognostic tool in heart failure. Measurement of BNP is currently only recommended in conjunction with standard clinical assessment and investigations. It remains largely a research tool while its role is being more specifically defined.

Nuclear imaging

If echocardiography imaging is inadequate to allow assessment of left ventricular function a radionucleotide ventriculogram may be performed, or if the patient proceeds to have cardiac catheterisation a contrast ventriculogram may be done.

Stress testing

If underlying coronary artery disease is suspected this may be investigated initially with stress testing. This is most commonly carried out by exercise testing with stress perfusion imaging and stress echocardiography is occasionally used. Stress echocardiography, most commonly using a dobutamine infusion, can be used to detect ischaemia as the cause of established left ventricular systolic dysfunction or to unmask reversible ischaemia-induced left ventricular systolic dysfunction. Exercise testing can also be used in heart failure to determine peak oxygen consumption (VO_2 max) as a prognostic marker and is a commonly employed investigation in research.

Cardiac catheterisation

It is important to exclude ischaemia as the cause of heart failure with left ventricular systolic dysfunction as revascularisation by percutaneous coronary intervention (PCI) or coronary artery bypass grafting (CABG) is known to improve prognosis.[9] Coronary angiography is therefore indicated when coronary artery disease is suspected or in some cases when no other cause for left ventricular systolic dysfunction has been identified. If there is evidence of significant valvular disease the severity of this should be further assessed by cardiac catheterisation.

Cardiac magnetic resonance imaging

Cardiac magnetic resonance imaging (MRI) is a powerful imaging technique but currently remains largely a research tool. Its potential role in the investigation and management of the heart failure patient is not yet clearly defined.

Summary

The assessment of a patient with heart failure should ideally involve the general practitioner, a cardiologist, and a heart failure nurse specialist. There is currently wide variation in the services provided across the UK with many heart failure patients managed by non-specialists and without the input of cardiologists or nurse specialists. With the growing burden of care for this patient population there is a need for well-directed use of healthcare resources such as the Glasgow Heart Failure Liaison Service. There is clearly room within heart failure service provision for this role to further expand, for example into supplementary prescribing, and as discussed in this chapter to involve a more comprehensive clinical assessment both in the home and potentially at nurse specialist clinics. For those nurses without this expertise, this would require a period of tuition and supervision to acquire the additional clinical skills described, local implementation, and the acquisition of evidence that it would be an effective addition to the service currently provided. However, as highlighted by the various case studies described in Appendix 2, an accurate assessment of the patient with heart failure remains the cornerstone of effective management.

References

1   McMurray JJ, Stewart S. Epidemiology, aetiology and prognosis of heart failure. *Heart* 2000;83:596–602.
2   Stewart S, MacIntyre K, Capewell S, McMurray JJ. Heart Failure and the ageing population: An increasing burden in the 21st Century? *Heart* 2003;89:49–53.
3   Stewart S, Jenkins A, Buchan S, Capewell S, McGuire A, McMurray JJ. The current cost of heart failure in the UK: An economic analysis. *Eur J Heart Fail* 2002;4:361–71.
4   Task force for the Diagnosis and Treatment of Chronic Heart Failure, European Society of Cardiology. Guidelines for the diagnosis and treatment of chronic heart failure. *Eur Heart J* 2001;22:1527–60.
5   Drexler H, Riede U, Munzel T, *et al*. Alterations of skeletal muscle in chronic heart failure. *Circulation* 1992;85:1751–9.

6   Goldberg LR, Piette JD, Walsh MN, *et al.* for the WHARF Investigators. Weight reduction trials. Randomized trial of a daily electronic home monitoring system in patients with advanced heart failure: the Weight Monitoring in Heart Failure (WHARF) trial. *Am Heart J* 2003;**146**:705–12.

7   Anker S, Ponikowski S, Varney S *et al.* Wasting as an independent risk factor for mortality in chronic heart failure. *Lancet* 1997;**349**:1050–3.

8   Byrne J, Davie AP, McMurray JJ. Clinical assessment and investigation of patients with suspected heart failure. In: Stewart S, Moser DM, Thompson DR, eds. *Caring for the heart failure patient*, London: Martin Dunitz, 2003.

9   Cleland J, Pennell DJ, Ray SG, *et al.* Myocardial viability as a determinant of the ejection fraction response to carvedilol in patients with heart failure (CHRISTMAS trial): randomised controlled trial. *Lancet* 2003;**362**:14–21.

8: Optimising the day to day management of patients with chronic heart failure

IONA MCKAY, SIMON STEWART

Introduction

Given a natural history[1] and prognostic impact[2] characterised by the complexity and heterogeneity of factors that can precipitate sudden episodes of acute decompensation requiring acute hospital care and even sudden death,[3] optimising the management of chronic heart failure is not an easy task. Add to that the complex array of individual responses that are precipitated and being confronted with a bewildering list of treatments and strategies whilst suffering from the debilitating effects of chronic disease (normally at an advanced age) makes the task seem even harder. Little wonder, therefore, that chronic heart failure has exposed the many flaws within current healthcare systems that have difficulty in dealing with highly prevalent chronic disease states which "demand" an intensive and individualised approach to improving health outcomes.

It was the undeniable inability of healthcare systems to manage a rising tide of heart failure that prompted the development of nurse-led strategies designed to apply not only the effective agents described in Chapter 2 in the "real world", but also adjunctive management strategies that, as a whole, provide clear benefits to the life situation of the patient.[4,5] The extensive research described in greater detail in Chapter 3 represents a fundamental truth that many clinicians are reluctant to advertise – there is no legitimate and widely available cure (or indeed "vaccine") for chronic heart failure. Although we have successfully improved heart failure related population survival rates in recent years,[6,7] we prolong rather than save lives in patients who are still likely to suffer and die from heart failure.[8]

A common wisdom in the face of the unknown or inevitable future is to take one day at a time. In attempting to optimise the management and treatment of chronic heart failure this is extremely good advice. It is on this basis that the Glasgow Heart Failure Liaison Service combines best pharmacological management with education strategies, practical advice, and caring support to enable patients to achieve the best quality of life, without offering unrealistic expectations of a cure. What the specialist heart failure nurses can offer patients is the chance to take greater control of their health to minimise the risk of hospitalisation and/or premature death within a caring environment.

In conjunction with the specific details provided in previous chapters (particularly Chapter 7, describing how to comprehensively assess the patient with heart failure), this chapter outlines the most important issues that need to be addressed when attempting to optimise the day to day management of heart failure. Naturally, given the predominantly home based service delivered by the specialist heart failure nurses in Glasgow, there is a strong focus on assessing and supporting patients in their own homes. However, the principles of care outlined in this chapter apply equally well to other forms of heart failure management, for example tele-health.

The role of post-discharge home visits

As described in more detail in Chapter 6, patients are admitted to the Glasgow service following an admission to hospital with an acute exacerbation of heart failure secondary to underlying left ventricular systolic dysfunction. Detailed information is gathered at this time from the hospital case notes before the patient goes home from hospital. Patients are then visited in their own homes within the first week of being discharged from hospital. As described in the supporting literature,[4,5,9–12] there is compelling evidence in support of home visits optimising the management of chronic heart failure irrespective of the type of follow-up thereafter. Specialist nurses who apply home based interventions in chronic heart failure unanimously agree that the first home visit is critical to understanding the patient's perspective of their illness, treatment, and overall life situation.

There are many preventable and often interrelated factors contributing to poorer outcomes among heart failure patients that can be addressed through careful assessment and non-pharmacological means. These potentially modifiable factors can be summarised as follows:

- inadequate or inappropriate medical treatment or adverse effects of prescribed treatment
- inadequate knowledge of chronic heart failure and prescribed treatment
- lack of motivation or inability to adhere to the treatment
- intentional non-compliance with prescribed treatment
- problems with caregivers or extended care facilities
- poor social support.[13–18]

As such, a cursory and task orientated home visit will not provide the type of detailed information required to identify the above issues and prepare effective plans to improve health outcomes in the longer term, nor the opportunity to implement early intervention to avoid morbidity and mortality in the short term. It is within this context that a comprehensive home visit designed to optimise the management of the patient suffering from chronic heart failure is often necessarily prolonged and often requires follow-up intervention to ensure that a complete picture of the patient (and where appropriate their main carer) is obtained. Only from a thorough home visit can a comprehensive plan to effectively address outstanding issues of concern be formulated. As described in Chapter 6 (see Table 6.1) the home visit, in conjunction with the detailed information collated prior to hospital discharge, enables the specialist heart failure nurse to determine the clinical stability of the patient, the prescribed treatment plan (both pharmacological and non-pharmacological) and the presence of potentially modifiable risk factors that may increase the probability of morbidity and mortality. Based on this information the nurse is able to formulate a flexible and individualised plan of action that will vary in intensity and duration based on the key issues identified. As such, there are seven key components of activity that comprise an effective and comprehensive home visit.

1. Holistic review of the patient's life situation

Immediately prior to visiting the patient it is important to review all information relating to their past and current medical history noting any additional information relevant to their health. Rather than immediately launching into a comprehensive review of the patient's clinical history and status, however, it is advisable to allow time for a general discussion with the patient (and carers if appropriate) to describe in general their life situation and how they perceive they came to be in their current state of health/illness. Such information provides important insights into how the patient (and carers) perceive and deal with the illness and how they generally interact with the health care system. In addition to crosschecking important health information, therefore, this overall review takes into consideration all the potential positive (for example community support/involvement) and negative (for example social or cultural isolation and poor relationships with health care providers) factors that may determine subsequent health outcomes.

One of the biggest problems overlooked in relation to the health of patients with heart failure is the psychological stress imposed by a chronic and debilitating condition that slowly drains them of their vitality and the ability to live as they would wish. Whilst it is clear that men and women approach these limitations differently,[19] it is clear from the literature and strong anecdotal evidence that anxiety and depression, with its associated effects on daily energy and motivation levels (particularly through sleep disturbance), is a major problem in patients suffering from chronic heart failure.[20-23] Without a careful and considered interview that adopts a holistic view of the patient and their life situation, the psychological health of the patient (and their carers[24] – see Appendix 3) may be overlooked.

2. Comprehensive clinical assessment

The value of carefully reviewing the patient's clinical history since hospital discharge coupled with a detailed clinical examination to detect signs of early clinical deterioration or factors that are likely to lead to such a scenario cannot be overstated. Figure 8.1 shows unexpectedly high rates of early clinical deterioration in a group of typical old and fragile patients (n = 88) visited in their home 7–14 days following discharge. Significantly, every patient had been reviewed by a general practitioner (most in a primary care clinic) in the week following their discharge.[25] Those who did display some form of clinical deterioration were more likely to be non-compliant with prescribed therapy and suffered higher morbidity and mortality rates in the six months following assessment despite active intervention.[25]

As described in much more detail in Chapter 7, there is a wealth of information that can be gained from a comprehensive physical assessment of the patient. Key areas of assessment include:

- functional status as determined by their New York Heart Association (NYHA) Classification status (see Table 7.4)
- overall activities of daily living (for example what are they able to achieve during the day?)
- lung sounds plus overall respiratory status
- heart sounds plus overall haemodynamic status (for example blood pressure and heart rate)
- peripheral integrity
- cognitive function
- hydration status.

These parameters provide the first clue as to whether the prescribed treatment and management plan is optimal in terms of maximising cardiac function and controlling the debilitating effects of the underlying heart failure and other potential conditions (for example myocardial ischaemia and chronic obstructive pulmonary disease). They also provide a comprehensive baseline with which to evaluate the effectiveness of any changes in the patient's management and/or assessing the severity of acute episodes of cardiac decompensation.

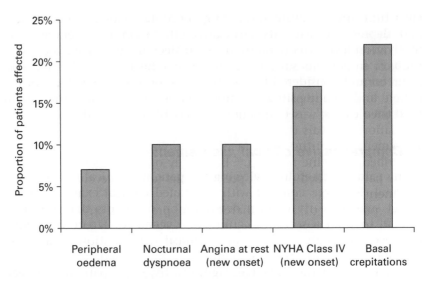

Figure 8.1 Early clinical deterioration detected in the home within 7 days of acute hospitalisation in 88 patients with chronic heart failure

3. Review of current treatment/management

As described in more detail in Chapter 9, the patient's current medication regimen should be checked to ensure that they are receiving a clinically proven pharmacological regimen and, conversely, are not prescribed or self-administering inappropriate therapy (for example a non-steroidal anti-inflammatory agent or "natural" therapies like St John's wort). If the patient has not been prescribed a regimen based on evidence-based medical guidelines, it is the responsibility of the heart failure nurse to address why this has occurred (for example was there a previous intolerance or adverse drug reaction or has it simply been overlooked?). It is common for an appropriate medication to be prescribed but in a sub-optimal dose and up-titration to a more clinically proven dose is, therefore, required. The heart failure nurses in the Glasgow service have the ability to up-titrate medication through the use of robust medical therapy guidelines. Medication changes can only be made once a full assessment of symptoms and blood chemistry analysis has been undertaken (see Chapter 9 for more details). Such assessment also extends to non-pharmacological strategies including fluid and salt management, exercise programmes, and secondary prevention (see below).

However, simply ensuring patients are prescribed the right pharmacological agents in the right doses addresses only a fraction of the issues surrounding optimal medication management. Adherence to long-term medical regimens of patients with heart failure is poor, with overall non-compliance rates ranging from 42%[26] to 64%.[27] In a study of elderly patients with heart failure, only 55% of the patients could correctly name what medication had been prescribed, 50% were unable to state the prescribed doses, and 64% could not account for what medication was to be taken, i.e. at what time of day and when in relation to meals the medication was to be taken. In their overall assessment the authors found that 73% were compliant with their prescribed medicine regimen.[28] In a study on digoxin use, only 10% of the patients filled enough prescriptions to have received adequate treatment.[29]

The problem of non-adherence to prescribed treatment also extends to other aspects of the treatment regimen like daily weighing, keeping a salt restricted diet, restricting fluid and alcohol intake and exercise. It seems difficult to change behaviour and to manage heart failure as expected by healthcare professionals. Strategies to enhance adherence include the patient but also integrate the role of physicians, nurses, other health care providers and organisations into the plan to ultimately improve patient outcomes. It is important to note that few studies have directly described the effect of a nurse-led heart failure intervention programme on treatment adherence[30-32] or readmissions arising from non-adherence to, or adverse effects of prescribed treatment.[33] However, it remains an important component of this type of intervention with strong anecdotal evidence of improved adherence rates and associated improvements in health outcomes.

It is extremely important, therefore, to assess the patient's level of adherence to prescribed treatment in addition to their knowledge concerning the purpose and possible adverse effects of these treatments. In practice, it is usually a caregiver who assumes responsibility for managing the therapeutic regimen on a day to day basis and any intervention (see below) is often directed to them. Figure 8.2 is a model of treatment adherence/knowledge based on patterns of medication management in a large cohort of chronically ill patients.[34] As such, it demonstrates that we need to consider the two components of treatment knowledge/awareness and adherence (represented on two different continuums) separately. For example, to the knowledgeable it would appear inadvisable to strictly adhere to prescribed high dose ACE inhibition when feeling increasingly dizzy, fatigued and, despite drinking reasonable amounts of water, finding no desire to void; yet such "blind adherence" is common and much less desirable than "reflective non-adherence" based on a sound knowledge of the risks and benefits of a prescribed regimen, a reasoned decision not to follow medical/nursing advice.

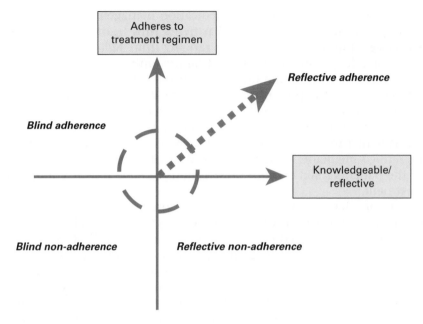

Figure 8.2 Model of treatment adherence and reflection

Ideally, most patients could be "trained" and motivated to practise "reflective adherence" to their treatment. However, in practical terms we often have to make do with applying strategies that provide a "safety net" to protect them against adverse effects and maximise potential benefits, knowing that rates of adherence and benefit are inversely related to the number of doses prescribed; i.e. the greater the potential for something to go wrong, the more likely it will go wrong! It is for this reason that many clinicians are now looking forward to the development of safe composite agents (for example combined ACE inhibition/β-blockade) in heart failure that will reduce the number of medications patients are forced to take.

4. Self-care/self-management

Although the increasing application of interactive telemonitoring devices is likely to provide greater surveillance in heart failure, it is clear that providing 24-hour health care is impossible and from a number of aspects undesirable for those living independently in the community. Instead, it is important that patients (and their caregivers) learn to live with the consequences of heart failure, which not only means complying with their prescribed treatment regimen (for example medication, diet, and exercise) but also actively monitoring their symptoms and seeking assistance when their condition deteriorates. The amount of time between the first awareness of symptoms and the arrival to the hospital (delay time) is often prolonged in patients with heart failure. Mean delays of 36 hours to one week before hospital admission are reported, with a median delay time of 72 hours.[35-36] Patients who reported with dyspnoea and oedema (the two most common symptoms of heart failure on admission) had delay times approximately twice as long a those who did not have these symptoms. It is more than likely that a large proportion of patients perceive these two chronic symptoms to be an integral and familiar component of their chronic condition and attempt to manage them at home before seeking acute assistance.[36]

It is imperative, therefore, for the specialist heart failure nurse to assist patients and carers to become more expert at self-managing their heart failure and learn when it is necessary to alter their treatment (for example diuretic titration based on increased weight) or take immediate action when a crisis appears imminent (for example increasing syncope attacks). As such, it has been demonstrated that a nurse-led heart failure management programme can positively affect these processes that probably affect patient outcomes.[37-39]

5. Education and counselling

As noted above, to ensure the optimum management of chronic heart failure with particular attention paid to minimising usually debilitating symptoms, it is necessary to encourage the patient wherever possible (remembering that many patients are unable) to assume an active role in their treatment and overall heart failure management. There are a number of key areas of management, other than that described in Chapter 9 in relation to prescribed pharmacotherapy, that can improve the health of the patient with heart failure. Based on the initial comprehensive assessment of the patient's clinical status and ability to self-care, these include the following.

Symptom monitoring and control

Patients and their carers need to be aware of the spectrum of symptoms commonly associated with heart failure and understand what should trigger a call for immediate/emergency nursing or medical assistance. For example, the box on p. 154 lists the questions concerning common symptoms associated with heart failure that will facilitate further discussion and establish the boundaries of "expected" versus clinically significant symptoms.

Key questions used to facilitate patient monitoring of heart failure symptoms

Breathlessness

Is your breathlessness worse than usual?
What types of activity provoke your feeling of breathlessness?
Do you wake at night feeling more breathless?
How many pillows did you use to sleep with last night?
Have you developed a cough recently?

Peripheral oedema

Do your legs show any sign of swelling?
If so, when does this swelling most commonly occur?
If you were to press your thumb into your lower leg does it leave an indent?
Do your shoes feel tight or your socks leave a clear mark during the day?
How far does the swelling extend (for example ankle, calf, knee, or thigh level)?

Fluctuations in weight

Do you know your "dry/optimal" weight?
When is the best time to monitor this?
What would you do if you noticed you had gained 2 kg or more over a few days?

Daily weight

A key component of symptom monitoring and control for many patients with heart failure (i.e. those with clear evidence of congestion) is fluid and dietary management. Where possible, determine the patient's ideal "dry" weight (when a patient who has had signs of fluid retention after diuretic treatment reaches a steady weight at which there are no further signs of fluid overload). Using this ideal weight as a goal, encourage patients to weigh themselves daily at the same time (usually morning in minimal clothes) and record their weight in the chart provided (usually in a patient diary). If the patient does not have a suitable set of scales, provide one. The patient should be advised that the best time for weighing is:

- every morning
- after going to toilet and
- before getting dressed and
- before breakfast.

Instruct patients (or family and carers where appropriate) that a steady weight gain over a number of days may indicate that they are retaining too much fluid. If this gain in weight is more than 2 kg (4 lb) over a few days they should contact their specialist heart failure nurse. Conversely, patients who lose a similar amount of weight over the same sort of period should also contact the nurse in case they have become dehydrated due to over-diuresis.

During episodes of fluid retention, the patient is encouraged to reduce fluid intake to 1·5 litres per day. Irrespective of the need for fluid restriction, patients should understand that an intake of over 2·5 litres per day should be avoided. It is important for the nurse to assist the patient in working out how much their usual cup, mug, or glass holds, and to suggest keeping a record of fluid intake until they become accustomed to how much they are allowed. Again this gives the patient a sense of control over their illness.

There is good evidence to suggest that, despite the proven beneficial effects of reducing sodium intake in even mild cases of heart failure, excessive sodium intake is a cause of episodes of acute decompensatory heart failure and non-responsiveness to diuretic therapy.[40–42] Although there is a paucity of evidence in terms of the optimal threshold for restricting sodium intake, an intake of around 2–3 grams per day is associated with clinical improvement and diuretic responsiveness.[40] Most patients, therefore, should be advised to avoid salt-rich foods and the addition of supplemental salt to food when cooking. Where appropriate, patients should be referred for specialist review and advice from a dietician (for example, patients with excessive fluid retention) to facilitate dietary knowledge and adherence.

Malnutrition and cardiac cachexia are common problems that contribute to debilitating symptoms of weakness and fatigue in addition to high levels of morbidity and mortality.[43–45] Cardiac cachexia is more likely to occur in the presence of anorexia, malabsorption, hypermetabolism, and poor dietary intake. The heart failure nurse should provide advice on choice of food and when to take medications. As above, support from a dietician may be necessary for further advice and for the introduction of nutritional supplements where required.

Medication adherence

As discussed, one of the main reasons for worsening heart failure symptoms is related to the issue of poor treatment adherence. For patients who have a good understanding of their illness and of their drug therapies, it may be possible for them to alter their own diuretic regime in response to a weight gain and worsening symptoms (see Chapter 9). A large proportion of patients, however, will need the support of the nurse before making a change to their medication regime.

Not surprisingly, the greater the number of prescribed doses, the greater the risk of non-adherence.[34] Weekly medication boxes (dosette box) are useful, but it is always helpful for the patient to have a separate prescription of diuretics in the house for times when symptoms are exacerbated. Adherence devices should, however, be reserved for those patients who are clearly unable to self-care and/or do not have a caregiver to support them. In these cases, the role of the community pharmacist may be particularly important.

There are a number of common problems that frequently arise in relation to non-adherence to, or inappropriate use of, prescribed pharmacotherapy. These include:

- having medications in the house that are no longer needed
- a lack of knowledge about prescribed drugs
- not knowing what dose should be taken
- unsure of what time the medication should be taken
- not receiving prescriptions on time and therefore running out of medication.

Communication with the patient's general practitioner, cardiologist, and pharmacist can be useful to assess the medication regimen and where possible to address significant problems associated with polypharmacy. Over the counter preparations that may cause a worsening of heart failure symptoms should be highlighted to the patient. The main drug group of concern are non-steroidal anti-inflammatory drugs as these can easily be bought over the counter. They may cause fluid retention and worsening renal failure.

Prevention

Respiratory infections are a major cause of avoidable heart failure related morbidity and mortality – particularly during winter months.[46,47] In view of this, all patients with heart failure should be encouraged to have an annual influenza immunisation and a single pneumococcal immunisation. The impact of this preventative step cannot be overstated given the dramatic (37%) reduction in hospital admissions for deteriorating heart failure in those patients immunised against influenza.[48] Limiting alcohol intake is also likely to reduce acute exacerbations given its negative impact on myocardial contractility and propensity to induce atrial fibrillation.[49,50]

It is often easy to overlook the factors that precipitated the development of heart failure, particularly in older patients. However, modifiable risk factors such as smoking, obesity, hypertension, hypercholesterolaemia, and sedentary behaviour (see below) are likely to directly or indirectly (for example by exacerbating the extent of myocardial ischaemia) aggravate underlying heart failure.[33] As such, efforts to proactively address these must be made.

Promoting exercise

A number of randomised trials have confirmed the benefits of both in-hospital and home exercise training programmes for heart failure.[51-53] Improved outcomes associated with these programmes include increased exercise capacity, decreased resting catecholamines, improved heart rate variability, and, most importantly, quality of life. However, the proportion of patients suitable for formal training programmes is likely to be fairly low (approximately 50%).[54] This does not mean, however, that the majority of patients should not be assessed and provided with a practical plan to promote their activity levels.

6. Establishing a practical long-term plan

Comprehensively assessing the current and future needs of the patient with heart failure is not easy. The box below and Figure 8.3 summarise the many factors to consider in assessing the patient in their own home and developing a long-term plan. As described in Chapter 6, the longer-term follow-up of the patient will depend on the combination of the following factors:

- level of assessed risk for poor health outcomes (for example high = advanced age, severe heart failure, treatment non-adherence, and/or poor psychosocial support)
- presence/absence of gold standard pharmacotherapy and non-pharmacologic strategies
- presence/absence of modifiable risk factors likely to exacerbate underlying heart failure.

Any plan of action has to involve the patient (and where appropriate caregivers) and the range of health care professionals involved in their ongoing management.

List of important components of a comprehensive home visit

Key assessments to be made where appropriate during the home visit

- assess the patient's heart failure status (for example, NYHA class, oedema, and sleeping pattern)
- assess the patient's general health status
- identify the available medical, nursing, and social support systems
- review the patient's medication to ensure they are receiving appropriate therapy in effective doses and adjust it according to medical therapy guidelines
- document the prescribed medication in the patient-held record book
- check and record the patient's blood pressure, heart rate, and weight
- check the blood chemistry
- update the patient's record book
- assess how much the patient understands about their condition and its treatment
- assess the patient's adherence to prescribed treatment
- update and reinforce the patient or carer with any information required

- provide additional educational support designed to increase the patient's knowledge of the prescribed medication (for example, the purpose, dosage, and potential side effects)
- ensure the patient has an adequate supply of medication
- educate the patient about daily weighing (for example, in the morning after going to the toilet, before having breakfast, and before getting dressed)
- provide additional education and advice concerning:
  - diet (including sodium intake, fluid intake, alcohol intake, weight reduction)
  - smoking
  - exercise
- advise the patient to have an annual influenza and single pneumococcal immunisation
- encourage the patient and the family or carers to be actively involved in managing and monitoring their own care
- plan the patient's future needs in accordance with the service guidelines and medical therapy guidelines
- communicate appropriate and effective information to all other health professionals involved in the patient's care.

7. Communicating and coordinating care

It is extremely important that the specialist heart failure nurse is able to utilise the information from a home visit and coordinate care accordingly. As noted in the first edition of this book, delineating the role of the specialist nurse in both the community and hospital setting is crucial to the long-term impact of the nurse intervention. Ideally, in the former this involves the following:

- management of the patient with chronic heart failure in the community in conjunction with the patient's general practitioner and cardiologist
- development of links with other community services, including community-based nurses, health visitors, community-based pharmacists, social services, palliative and emergency care services.

In relation to the latter it involves the following:

- identifying hospitalised patients with chronic heart failure who meet the criteria for post-discharge specialist nurse management
- promoting the service with staff in whatever speciality or general units chronic heart failure patients are usually managed in (medical, cardiology, coronary care, and geriatric units)
- liaising with ward staff regarding patient referral to the service and timing of discharge from hospital
- accessing cardiology expertise for advice and clinical support
- developing links with other important services (echocardiography, biochemistry, haematology, pharmacy, cardiac rehabilitation, and palliative care).

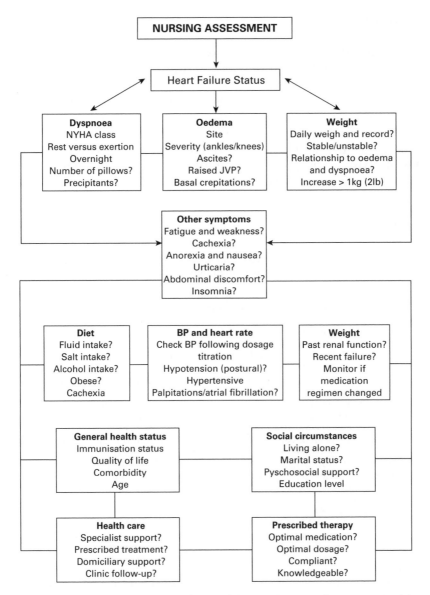

Figure 8.3 Nursing assessment of heart failure – the many factors to consider

The specialist heart failure nurse is responsible for creating a constructive and harmonious relationship with other healthcare professionals for the benefit of the patient. As such they often represent the "human face" of health care and assist the patient to navigate through the often bewildering complexities and idiosyncrasies of the overall healthcare system.

Summary

The crucial importance of assessing patients in their own home cannot be overstated as it provides a critical platform for establishing the presence of previously unknown factors likely to positively or negatively influence subsequent health outcomes. The complexity of assessment and planning required to achieve the optimal management of heart failure also cannot be overstated. However, with clear guidelines and planning, applied on an individualised and flexible basis, it is possible to improve health outcomes in heart failure on a day to day basis.

References

1   Peeters A, Mamun AA, Willekens F, Bonneux L. A cardiovascular life history: A life course analysis of the original Framingham Heart Study cohort. *Eur Heart J* 2002;**23**:458–66.

2   Stewart S, MacIntyre K, Hole DJ, Capewell S, McMurray JJ. More 'malignant' than cancer? Five-year survival following a first admission for heart failure. *Eur J Heart Fail* 2001;**3**:315–22.

3   Bennett SJ, Huster GA, Baker SL, *et al*. Characterization of the precipitants of hospitalization for heart failure decompensation. *Am J Crit Care* 1998;**7**:168–74.

4   McMurray JJ, Stewart S. Nurse-led multidisciplinary intervention in chronic heart failure. *Heart* 1998;**80**:430–1.

5   Rich MW. Heart failure disease management: a critical review. *J Cardiac Fail* 1999;**5**:64–75.

6   MacIntyre K, Capewell S, Stewart S, *et al*. Evidence of improving prognosis in heart failure: trends in case-fatality in 66547 patients hospitalized between 1986 and 1995. *Circulation* 2000;**102**:1126–31.

7   Levy D, Kenchaiah S, Larson MG, *et al*. Long-term trends in the incidence of and survival with heart failure. *N Engl J Med* 2002;**347**:1397–402.

8   Stewart S, McMurray JJ. Palliative care for heart failure. *BMJ* 2002;**325**:915–6.

9   Stewart S, Marley JE, Horowitz JD. Effects of a multidisciplinary, home-based intervention on unplanned readmissions and survival among patients with chronic congestive heart failure: a randomised controlled study. *Lancet* 1999;**354**:1077–83.

10 Blue L, Lang E, McMurray JJ, *et al*. Randomised controlled trial of specialist nurse intervention in heart failure. *BMJ* 2001;**323**:715–18.

11 Stewart S, Horowitz JD. Home-based intervention in congestive heart failure: long-term implications on readmission and survival. *Circulation* 2002;**105**:2861–6.

12 Thompson DR, Roebuck A, Stewart S. Effects of a nurse-led, clinic and home-based intervention on recurrent hospital use in chronic heart failure. *Eur Heart J* 2003; **24**:485.

13 Wolinski FD, Smith DM, Stump TE, Everhoge JM, Lubitz RM. The sequelae of hospitalisation for congestive heart failure among older adults. *J Am Geriatr Soc* 1997;**45**:558–63.

14 Krumholz HM, Parent EM, Tu N, *et al*. Readmission after hospitalisation for congestive heart failure among Medicare beneficiaries. *Arch Intern Med* 1997;**157**:99–104.

15 Vinson JM, Rich MW, Sperry JC. Early readmission of elderly patients with congestive heart failure. *J Am Geriatr Soc* 1990;**38**:1290–5.

16 Happ MB, Naylor MD, Roe-Prior P. Factors contributing to rehospitalization of elderly patients with heart failure. *J Cardiovasc Nurs* 1997;**11**:75–84.

17 Michalsen A, Konig G, Thimme W. Preventable causative factors leading to hospital admission with decompensated heart failure. *Heart* 1998;**80**:437–41.

18 Tsuyuki RT, McKelvie RS, Arnold JM, *et al.* Acute precipitants of congestive heart failure exacerbations. *Arch Intern Med* 2001;**161**:2337–42.

19 Murberg TA, Bru E, Aarsland T, Svebak S. Functional status and depression among men and women with congestive heart failure. *Int J Psychiatry Med* 1998; **28**:273–91.

20 Levenson JW, McCarthy EP, Lynn J, Davis RB, Phillips RS. The last six months of life for patients with congestive heart failure. *J Am Geriatr Soc* 2000;**48**:S101–9.

21 Krumholz HM, Phillips RS, Hamel MB, *et al.* Resuscitation preferences among patients with severe congestive heart failure: results from the SUPPORT project. *Circulation* 1998;**98**:648–55.

22 Koenig HG. Depression in hospitalised older patients with congestive heart failure. *Gen Hosp Psych* 1998;**20**:29–43.

23 Freedland KE, Carney RM, Rich MW, *et al.* Depression in elderly patients with congestive heart failure. *Geriatr Psych* 1991;**24**:59–71.

24 Luttik M, Jaarsma T, Van Veldhuisen DJ. Quality of life of caregivers is worse compared to patients with congestive heart failure. *Eur Heart J* 2003;**24**:64.

25 Stewart S, Horowitz JD. Detecting early clinical deterioration in chronic heart failure patients post acute hospitalisation – a critical component of multidisciplinary, home-based intervention? *Eur J Heart Fail* 2002;**4**:345–51.

26 Tsuyuki RT, McKelvie RS, Arnold JM, *et al.* Acute precipitants of congestive heart failure exacerbations. *Arch Intern Med* 2001;**161**:2337–42.

27 Ghali JK, Kadakia S, Cooper R, Ferlinz J. Precipitating factors leading to decompensation of heart failure. Traits among urban blacks. *Arch Intern Med* 1988;**148**:2013–7.

28 Cline CM, Bjorck-Linne AK, Israelsson BY, Willenheimer RB, Erhardt LR. Non-compliance and knowledge of prescribed medication in elderly patients with heart failure. *Eur J Heart Fail* 1999;**1**:145–9.

29 Monane M, Bohn RL, Gurwitz JH, Glynn RJ, Avorn J. Noncompliance with congestive heart failure therapy in the elderly. *Arch Intern Med* 1994;**154**:433–7.

30 Riegel B, Carlson B. Facilitators and barriers to heart failure self-care. *Patient Educ Couns* 2002;**46**:287–95.

31 Rich MW, Gray DB, Beckham V, Wittenberg C, Luther P. Effect of a multidisciplinary intervention on medication compliance in elderly patients with congestive heart failure. *Am J Med* 1996;**101**:270–6.

32 Krumholz HM, Amatruda J, Smith GL, *et al.* Randomized trial of an education and support intervention to prevent readmission of patients with heart failure. *J Am Coll Cardiol* 2002;**39**:83–9.

33 Moser DK, Lennie TA, Doering LV. Non-pharmacologic management of heart failure. In: Stewart S, Moser DK, Thompson DR, eds. *Caring for heart failure.* London: Martin Dunitz, 2004.

34 Stewart S, Pearson S. Uncovering a multitude of sins: medication management in the home post acute hospitalisation among the chronically ill. *Aust NZ J Med* 1999;**29**:220–7.

35 Friedman MM. Older adults' symptoms and their duration before hospitalization for heart failure. *Heart Lung* 1997;**26**:169–76.

36 Evangelista LS, Dracup K, Doering LV. Treatment-seeking delays in heart failure patients. *J Heart Lung Transplant* 2000;**19**:932–8.

37 Jaarsma T, Halfens R, Huijer Abu-Saad H, *et al.* Effects of education and support on self-care and resource utilization in patients with heart failure. *Eur Heart J* 1999;**20**:673–82.

38 Riegel B, Carlson B, Glaser O, Hoaglund P. Which patients with heart failure respond best to multidisciplinary disease management. *J Card Fail* 2000;**6**: 290–9.

39 Strömberg A, Martensson J, Fridlund B, Levin LA, Karlsson JE, Dahlstrom U. Nurse-led heart failure clinics improve survival and self-care behaviour in patients with heart failure: results from a prospective, randomised trial. *Eur Heart J* 2003;**24**: 1014–23.

40 Cody RJ, Pickworth KK. Approaches to diuretic therapy and electrolyte imbalance in congestive heart failure. *Cardiol Clin* 1994;**12**:37–50.

41 Kramer BK, Schweda F, Riegger GA. Diuretic treatment and diuretic resistance in heart failure. *Am J Med* 1999;**106**:90–6.

42 Tang WH, Francis GS. Polypharmacy of heart failure. Creating a rational pharmacotherapeutic protocol. *Cardiol Clin* 2001;**19**:583–96.

43 Anker SD, Coats AJ. Cachexia in heart failure is bad for you. *Eur Heart J* 1998; **19**:191–3.

44 Anker SD, Coats AJ. Cardiac cachexia: a syndrome with impaired survival and immune and neuroendocrine activation. *Chest* 1999;**115**:836–47.

45 Anker SD, Ponikowski P, Varney S, *et al*. Wasting as independent risk factor for mortality in chronic heart failure. *Lancet* 1997;**349**:1050–3.

46 Stewart S, McIntyre K, Capewell S, McMurray JJ. Heart failure in a cold climate: Seasonal variation in heart failure-related morbidity and mortality. *J Am Coll Cardiol* 2002;**39**:760–6.

47 Boulay F, Berthier F, Sisteron O, Gendreike Y, Gibelin P. Seasonal variation in chronic heart failure hospitalizations and mortality in France. *Circulation* 1999;**100**:280–6.

48 Nichol KL, Margolis KL, Wuorenma J, Von Sternberg TL. The efficacy and cost effectiveness of vaccination against influenza among elderly persons living in the community. *N Engl J Med* 1994;**331**:778–84.

49 Ghali JK, Kadakia S, Cooper R, Ferlinz J. Precipitating factors leading to decompensation of heart failure. Traits among urban blacks. *Arch Intern Med* 1988;**9**:2013–6.

50 Opasich C, Febo O, Riccardi PG, *et al*. Concomitant factors of decompensation in chronic heart failure. *Am J Cardiol* 1996;**78**:354–7.

51 Sullivan MJ, Higginbotham MB, Cobb FR. Exercise training in patients with severe left ventricular dysfunction. Hemodynamic and metabolic effects. *Circulation* 1988; **78**:506–15.

52 European Heart Training Working Group. Experience from controlled trials of physical training in chronic heart failure: protocol and patient factors in effectiveness in the improvement in exercise tolerance. *Eur Heart J* 1998;**19**:466–75.

53 Belardinelli R, Georgiou D, Cianci G, Purcaro A. Randomized, controlled trial of long-term moderate exercise training in chronic heart failure: effects on functional capacity, quality of life, and clinical outcome. *Circulation* 1999;**99**:1173–82.

54 Gottlieb SS, Fisher ML, Freudenberger R, *et al*. Effects of exercise training on peak performance and quality of life in congestive heart failure patients. *J Card Fail* 1999;**5**:188–94.

9: Pharmacological treatment for chronic heart failure: a specialist nurse perspective

YVONNE MILLERICK

Introduction

As described in greater detail in Chapter 2, gold standard pharmacological treatment of chronic heart failure secondary to left ventricular systolic dysfunction includes specifically recommended doses of an angiotensin converting enzyme (ACE) inhibitor and a β-blocker in addition to the combination of a diuretic, spironolactone, and digoxin.[1,2] Given the results of the CHARM-Added and CHARM-Alternative trials,[3–5] angiotensin receptor blockers are likely to be added to this list in some if not the majority of patients (i.e. those who are unable to tolerate an ACE inhibitor or alternatively those on maximal therapy in whom more complete inhibition of angiotensin II would provide greater control of refractory symptoms).

Applying gold standard pharmacotherapy in the same way as that applied in clinical trials is never easy when the profile of patients in the "real world" differs so markedly from trial cohorts – particularly when there is limited time to deal with more complex clinical issues surrounding up-titration and adverse effects.[6,7] The key advantage of specialist nurse-led intervention in heart failure is the availability of dedicated and qualified nurses who can individually tailor gold standard pharmacotherapy according to the clinical profile and needs of the patient. As discussed in Chapter 8, the specialist nurse is in a unique position to determine the factors likely to positively and negatively affect patient outcomes. Such considerations are important when applying a complex treatment regimen.

Chapter 2 represents a more detailed review (with an extensive list of references) of the evidence in support of the main pharmacological agents described here. As such, this chapter is designed to outline the pharmacological management of patients with chronic heart failure (predominantly secondary to left ventricular systolic dysfunction) from a pragmatic perspective and within the scope of practice of the specialist heart failure nurse. Further evidence of this pragmatic approach can be found in the case studies described in Appendix 2.

Disclaimer. It is important to note that the information in this chapter should not be substituted for specifically designed guidelines and protocols that have been reviewed and approved by a cardiologist and a local healthcare authority. Loosely based on the guidelines applied within the Glasgow Heart Failure Liaison Service, the information and advice contained herein are presented for educational purposes only.

Aims of heart failure treatment

The main aims of pharmacological intervention in chronic heart failure should be to ameliorate symptoms, optimise appropriate drug therapy whilst minimising inappropriate drug therapy in order to reduce inappropriate hospital admissions, prolong survival, and, perhaps most importantly, improve the patient's quality of life.

Drugs regularly used to treat heart failure

The following pharmacological agents are most commonly used in the treatment of chronic heart failure:

- diuretics
- ACE inhibitors
- β-blockers
- spironolactone
- digoxin
- angiotensin receptor blockers
- nitrates and hydralazine.[1,2,8]

There is little doubt that various combinations of these drugs improve patient symptoms and have contributed to recent improvements in population survival rates, and will continue to do so as the impact of newer agents accumulates.[9] As noted in Chapter 2, the majority of evidence in favour of these agents relates to the management of patients with underlying left ventricular systolic dysfunction.

Diuretics

Diuretic therapy continues to play a vital role in the management of both acute and chronic heart failure by providing symptomatic relief of breathlessness and peripheral oedema. On reviewing the patient the nurse should be thinking, is the diuretic dose sufficient to achieve a "dry" weight (in other words is the patient free from peripheral oedema, a raised jugular venous pressure, and signs of pulmonary congestion)? Everyday experience shows us that diuretics can improve symptoms and this can lead to increased functional activity and therefore improved quality of life. There are three main groups of diuretics: loop, thiazides, and potassium sparing diuretics.

Loop diuretics increase water excretion by inhibiting the reabsorption of sodium chloride from the ascending Loop of Henle. Diuresis can begin 1–2 hours following oral administration and their effects can persist for up to 4–6 hours thereafter.

Thiazides increase sodium, water, and potassium excretion at the beginning of the distal convoluted tubule. Diuresis can begin 1–2 hours following oral administration; however, in contrast to loop diuretics, the diuresis can continue for up to 12–24 hours.

Potassium sparing diuretics (with the exception of spironolactone) are not commonly used to treat heart failure. They inhibit sodium reabsorption and conserve potassium. It is for this reason that patients who are on an ACE inhibitor and potassium sparing therapy should be monitored closely for hyperkalaemia.

Key clinical issues

Problems associated with diuretics usually occur as a result of over treatment leading to dehydration. Dehydration can manifest itself in a number of different ways and some of the most common symptoms include:

- thirst
- dizziness
- fatigue
- light-headedness
- gout
- a feeling of being "washed out".

Other subtle changes can often be observed by the nurse such as flaky skin or skin turgor (an abnormality in the skin's ability to change shape and return to normal). The skin, usually on the back of the hand, is grasped between two fingers and is held for a few seconds then released (see Figure 9.1). Skin with normal turgor will return to its normal position immediately. Patient's skin with decreased turgor does not revert to its normal position for some time.[10]

There are other more subtle changes in the patient's condition that may alert the nurse to the fact that they have become dehydrated. For example, the patient may develop hypotension when usually normotensive, venepuncture may prove to be difficult

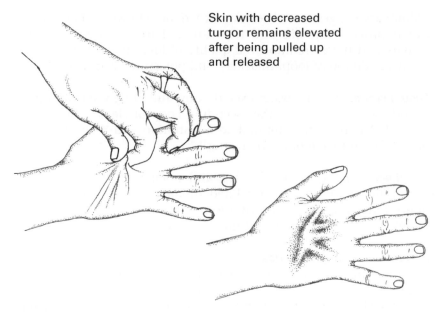

Skin with decreased turgor remains elevated after being pulled up and released

Figure 9.1 Assessing skin turgor

due to hypovolaemia, and the patient may express difficulty in passing urine or complain of constipation. Other symptoms, particularly in the elderly, can be very non-specific and include confusion, impaired mobility, falls, and the development of incontinence.

Non-adherence to diuretic therapy

Diuretics continue to be a major inconvenience for patients and can lead to treatment non-adherence. It is for this reason that the nurse should spend time encouraging the patient to adopt a flexible diuretic regime. The patient should be made aware that their prescribed diuretic need not be taken at the same time each day. Postponing or adjusting the time of the diuretic to suit a daily routine will lead to better symptom control and overall drug adherence.

Therapeutic monitoring

Close monitoring of blood chemistry is necessary following initiation of a diuretic or within one week of a dosage increment. The nurse should be alerted to changes that suggest the patient is dehydrated. These changes may include elevated levels of urea and

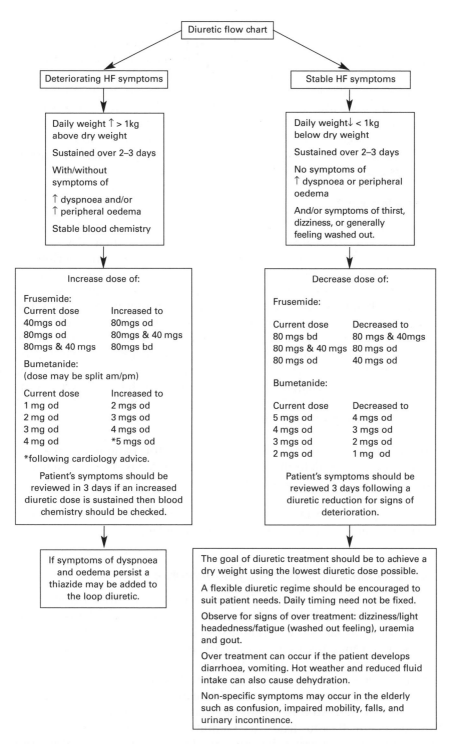

Figure 9.2 Guidance on diuretic treatment in chronic heart failure

creatinine, leading to hyperkalaemia, hypokaleamia, and/or hyponatraemia. Baseline blood chemistry must always be checked by the nurse and following any sustained increase in diuretic dose (> 1 week). If the urea > 20 mmol/l (or ↑ by 10 mmol/l), and/or creatinine increases to > 300 micromol/l (or ↑ by > 100 micromol/l), and/or the potassium decreases to < 3·5 micromol/l or below, the nurse should contact a cardiologist or other appropriate physician for advice. If the patient is able to sustain their "dry weight" (see above) for a prolonged period (for example greater than one month) and/or appears dehydrated then the diuretic dose should be reduced.

Dose adjustment

Increasing the diuretic dose is necessary if the patient shows a sustained weight gain of 1 kg or more above their dry weight associated with symptoms of increasing dyspnoea and peripheral oedema for more than three consecutive days. Usually, dose adjustment should only occur in single incremental doses (for example if the patient is taking 40 mg of furosemide once daily the dose should be increased to 80 mg once daily). Or alternatively, if the patient is taking 1 mg once daily of bumetanide, the dose should be increased to 2 mg once daily. Initially the increased dose should be maintained for three days only. If a dry weight is reached, the patient can revert to the original lower diuretic dose. If, however, symptoms persist specialist (for example cardiology) advice should be sought before increasing the dose further.

Decreasing a diuretic should only occur if the patient has reached their individually determined dry weight and has no overt signs of fluid overload. Dosage should be adjusted in the same increments as used for increasing doses. It is important to remember that the major aim is to prescribe the smallest dose of diuretic necessary to keep the patient clinically stable and euvolaemic (see Figure 9.2).

Angiotensin converting enzyme inhibitors

As discussed in Chapter 2, large randomised controlled trials have demonstrated that ACE inhibitors improve survival in patients with all grades of heart failure. When added to diuretic therapy they improve signs, symptoms, and exercise capacity, reduce hospital admission due to deteriorating heart failure, and slow the natural progression from mild to severe symptoms indicative of this syndrome.[1,2,8]

Patients with heart failure have increased activity from the renin–angiotensin–aldosterone system that leads to high levels of angiontensin II and leads to sodium and water retention. ACE inhibitors are effective because of their ability to inhibit the

Table 9.1 Titration of ACE inhibitor therapy

ACE inhibitor	Target dose	Increments at weekly intervals
Captopril	50 mg tid	12·5 – 25 mg
Enalapril	20 mg bd	2·5 – 5 mg
Ramipril	5 mg bd	2·5 mg
Lisinopril	35 mg od	2·5 – 5 mg

production of angiotensin II. They therefore reduce peripheral vascular resistance and increase the vasodilatory effects of bradykinin. Bradykinin is thought to be responsible for some of the negative effects from ACE inhibitors such as the irritable cough, hypotension and renal impairment.[10]

In the absence of specific contraindications such as symptomatic hypotension and renal impairment, all patients with heart failure secondary to left ventricular systolic dysfunction should be considered for treatment with an ACE inhibitor.

Prior to introducing ACE inhibitor therapy, the nurse should ensure that all potassium supplements and potassium sparing diuretics are stopped. Baseline blood chemistry must be checked and observed for elevated levels of creatinine > 200 micromol/l, urea > 15 mmol/l, hyperkalaemia, and hyponatraemia. Systolic blood pressure should also be above 90 mmHg systolic. If the patient has asymptomatic hypotension (< 90 mmHg systolic) medical advice should always be sought before initiating or increasing ACE inhibitor therapy.

Dose adjustment

ACE inhibitor therapy should always be started at the lowest dose and increased by titration to a maximum tolerated dose. There should be at least one week between each dosage increment and there should be close monitoring to detect possible adverse effects. In the absence of symptomatic hypotension and renal impairment the increments shown in Table 9.1 can be routinely applied.

Key clinical issues

As noted, a bradykinin related cough is commonly associated with this class of agent, although, if tolerated, it is not an indication for stopping treatment. Only when the cough is completely intolerable and is clearly related to the ACE inhibitor therapy should consideration be given to substituting it with an angiotensin receptor blocker.

Hypoperfusion (cerebral and renal) can be a problem although it is often possible to reverse by reducing the patient's diuretic dose provided there is no evidence of sodium and water retention.

Consideration should also be given to stopping other pharmacological agents that have no value in heart failure but could be contributing to the adverse symptoms (for example nitrates unless indicated for angina pectoris). Other less common side effects include a rash (that may or may not be associated with pruritis), nausea, vomiting, abdominal pain, and headache.

Therapeutic monitoring

Following any initiation or dosage change the patient should be checked within one week for signs of symptomatic hypotension, intolerable cough, and renal impairment. Changes in blood chemistry such as hyperkalaemia of > 5·5 micromol/l, elevated urea > 20 mmol/l, creatinine levels > 300 micromol/l, and hyponatraemia of < 133 micromol/l are significant and should be discussed with the treating physician (see Figure 9.3).

Beta-blockers

Beta-blockers have rapidly become part of the gold standard treatment of heart failure in combination with diuretics and ACE inhibitor therapy. Large-scale clinical trials have demonstrated that β-blockers reduce mortality and morbidity, improve left ventricular function and symptoms, and reduce hospital admissions for deteriorating heart failure in patients with mild to severe heart failure associated with left ventricular systolic dysfunction.[1,2,8]

Key clinical issues

Treatment should be considered for patients who are clinically stable and have not had a diuretic adjustment in the past two weeks or a hospital admission for deteriorating heart failure in the past month. They should already be receiving standard treatment with a diuretic, ACE inhibitor, and/or digoxin.

A cardiologist/physician should review all patients before commencing a β-blocker. The only absolute contraindication to β-blocker therapy is true bronchial reactive asthma. All other patients should be screened for deteriorating heart failure symptoms, symptomatic hypotension (systolic blood pressure < 90 mmHg), heart block and sick sinus syndrome. The clinical management of those patients who demonstrate asymptomatic hypotension and/or a bradycardia of less than 55 bpm should be discussed with a cardiologist before initiating or increasing β-blocker therapy. Other considerations that may deter patients from tolerating β-blocker therapy are those who suffer from peripheral vascular disease. From experience this patient group may only tolerate a small dose of β-blocker – if at all.

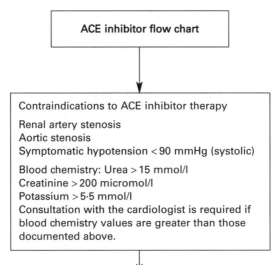

ACE inhibitor flow chart

Contraindications to ACE inhibitor therapy

Renal artery stenosis
Aortic stenosis
Symptomatic hypotension < 90 mmHg (systolic)

Blood chemistry: Urea > 15 mmol/l
Creatinine > 200 micromol/l
Potassium > 5·5 mmol/l
Consultation with the cardiologist is required if
blood chemistry values are greater than those
documented above.

ACE inhibitor therapy should always be started at the lowest dose
and gradually increased at **weekly intervals** until a maximum
tolerated or target dose is reached.

Initiation away from hospital environment should be supported with
advice to prevent symptomatic hypotension that can occur following
the first dose. Simple instruction such as advising the patient to take
the ACE inhibitor at a different time from their other medication is
often enough.

	Start Dose	Increments	Target
Captopril	6·25mg	12·5mg	50mg tid
Enalapril	2·5mg	2·5mg	10–20mg bd
Ramipril	1·25mg	2·5mg	5mg bd
Lisinopril	2·5mg	2·5mg	10–35mg od

These are only some examples of the ACE inhibitor therapies used

Monitoring

Patient's BP, blood chemistry, and symptoms should be reviewed within 1
week of initiation or titration of ACE inhibitor therapy.
In the absence of any adverse effects titration can continue at weekly intervals
until the maximum or target dose is reached.

Once patient has reached target dose, blood chemistry should be reviewed at
6 monthly intervals long term.

If adverse effects do occur further titration should be postponed until patient
stabilises. Cardiologist should be advised and if necessary the ACE inhibitor
dose should be reduced or stopped temporarily to allow symptoms to resolve.

In some instances such as an intolerant cough the patient may need to change
to angiotensin II receptor antagonist.

Figure 9.3 Guidance on ACE inhibitor treatment in chronic heart failure

Deteriorating heart failure symptoms The nurse should advise the patient that following initiation or increased dose of a β-blocker symptoms of increasing dyspnoea might develop on the third or fourth day. However, by temporarily increasing their diuretic dose symptoms will usually resolve. Before a dose change the nurse must be satisfied that the patient's heart failure symptoms are stable and that both the blood pressure and heart rate are satisfactory. If the heart failure symptoms fail to respond to the increase in diuretic therapy it may be necessary to reduce or stop the β-blocker dose until such times as the patient's symptoms stabilise.

Hypotension There are many possible causes of hypotension. The nurse needs to determine if the patient has asymptomatic hypotension and if so this should be monitored closely. If however the patient has symptomatic hypotension then the following measures should be considered.

- If the patient is euvolaemic/dehydrated reduce their diuretic dose.
- Discontinue other hypotensive drugs of no value in heart failure.
- Consider temporarily decreasing the ACE inhibitor dose.

If symptomatic hypotension persists despite these measures then the nurse should discuss with a cardiologist reducing the dosage and/or stopping the β-blocker.

Bradycardia If a patient's heart rate is < 55 bpm and they are asymptomatic, the β-blocker dose should be reduced. Alternatively, if the patient is symptomatic treatment should be stopped immediately and a further review should take place in one week. If the bradycardia persists consideration should be given to reducing or stopping other rate controlling drugs such as digoxin, diltiazem, and amiodarone provided the cardiologist is in full agreement. If the patient's heart rate is < 45 bpm the β-blocker should be stopped immediately and a 12-lead ECG obtained. The patient's cardiologist/specialist physician should be alerted to the possibility of β-blocker induced heart block or sick sinus syndrome.

Dosage adjustment

Figure 9.4 shows the dosage adjustment for two of the most commonly used β-blockers (carvedilol and bisoprolol). Not surprisingly, with additional experience in using β-blockers, there is increasing evidence of their prescription and up-titration in the primary care setting as opposed to the hospital setting. This closely parallels the experience of ACE inhibition. However, at this stage of the application of β-blockers (particularly in older patients receiving "triple"

Beta-blocker flow chart

Beta-blockers are well tolerated in heart failure and should be considered for all patients with left ventricular systolic dysfunction who do not have any contraindications.

Contraindications
True bronchial reactive asthma

Pre-initiation checks

Clinically stable
Heart rate > 55 beats per minute and systolic blood pressure > 90 mmHg
No contraindications to β-blockade

Carvedilol	Bisoprolol
(License states)	(License states)
Initiated and titrated under the supervision of a hospital physician	Initiated and titrated by a physician experienced in the treatment of heart failure

Titration

Week 1	3·125 mg bd
Week 3	6·25 mg bd
Week 5	12·5 mg bd
Week 7	25 mg bd
Week 9	*50 mg bd

*If weight > 85 kg
Titration should be tailored to suit individual needs of patients. This may mean that titration schedules are slightly variable.

Titration

Week 1	1·25 mg od
Week 2	2·5 mg od
Week 3	3·75 mg od
Week 4	5 mg od
Week 8	7·5 mg od
Week 11	10 mg od

Titration should be tailored to suit individual needs of patients. This may mean that titration schedules are slightly variable.

Management of adverse effects

Worsening heart failure	Symptomatic hypotension	Excessive bradycardia
• dyspnoea • weight • peripheral oedema ↑ Diuretic dose for 3 days Symptoms resolve, revert to lower diuretic dose and continue with β-blocker. Symptoms persist, consider reducing or stopping the β-blocker dose temporarily. Wait 4 weeks before attempting to up-titrate or reinitiate β-blocker.	• Consider over-diuresis and ↓ diuretic dose • If symptoms persist consider reducing or stopping other hypotensive causing drugs of no value in heart failure. • Consider temporarily reducing the ACE inhibitor dose • Reduce or stop the β-blocker. Wait 4 weeks before before attempting to up-titrate or reinitiate β-blocker therapy.	• Heart rate < 55 beats per min • If symptomatic consider stopping β-blocker • Asymptomatic revert to the lower β-blocker dose • Consider stopping or reducing other rate controlling drugs Review within 1 week, alert cardiologist if bradycardia persists • Heart rate < 45 beats per minute • Stop β-blocker and arrange a 12-lead ECG, inform the cardiologist • Look for signs of heart block or sick sinus syndrome.

Blood pressure, heart rate, and heart failure status should be reviewed in patients pre and post dose change to help identify and treat possible adverse effects.

Figure 9.4 Guidance on β-blocker treatment in chronic heart failure

neurohormonal therapy) caution is required to achieve the following targets with dosage adjustments occurring at least 14 days apart:

- carvedilol: start at 3·125 mg bd until a target dose of 25 mg bd is reached by week 7 or 50 mg at week 9 if the patient is > 85 kg.
- bisoprolol: start at 1·25 mg once daily until a target dose of 10 mg is reached by week 12.

Spironolactone

Spironolactone is a potassium sparing diuretic that inhibits the renin–angiotensin system. It potentiates the action of loop and/or thiazide diuretics by antagonising aldosterone. The Randomised Aldactone Evaluation Study (RALES) was stopped prematurely because of a significant reduction in mortality.

Patients who continue to have signs of persistent sodium and water retention despite treatment with diuretics, ACE inhibition, and/or digoxin should be considered for treatment with low dose spironolactone. Initiation should always be discussed with the patient's cardiologist.[1,2,8]

Dose

The RALES study dose was 25 mg once daily. To date there has been no further evidence to support the use of larger doses in heart failure patients. From experience however it is not uncommon for patients who have difficulty tolerating the 25 mg to be maintained on a daily dose of 12·5 mg without adverse effect and with improved heart failure status.

Key clinical issues

Spironolactone can cause many problems and it is for this reason that many patients cannot tolerate it on a daily basis. Common effects are gastrointestinal disturbances such as nausea, vomiting, and/or diarrhoea. Should these symptoms occur the spironolactone must be stopped immediately. Other symptoms include gynaecomastia that can often be very painful and therefore intolerable for patients. The nurse should be observing for signs of hyponatraemia and hyperkalaemia, again common side effects of this treatment.

Therapeutic monitoring

The nurse specialist should ensure that baseline blood chemistry has been checked before initiation of this line of treatment. Contra-indications to spironolactone include serum creatinine level greater than 200 micromol/l, serum urea greater than 11 micromol/l, and serum potassium greater than 4·5 micromol/l. If the patient is on potassium sparing diuretics these should be substituted with appropriate potassium losing diuretics and all potassium supplements should be discontinued two weeks before starting spironolactone.

Following initiation of spironolactone, blood chemistry must be checked one week, two weeks, and four weeks of treatment. Further checks should be every four weeks for three months, every three months for one year, and then every six months thereafter. If the patient complains of diarrhoea and vomiting leading to water and sodium depletion, once again the spironolactone should be stopped immediately.

Treatment should also be discontinued if blood chemistry deteriorates and the following parameters are breached:

- serum creatinine increases to 250 micromol/l or by 25% from baseline (for example 80 to 100 micromol/l)
- urea increases to greater than 18 micromol/l or by 50% from baseline (for example 8 to 12 micromol/l)
- potassium increases to greater than 5·5 micromol/l.

The specialist nurse should also be observing for signs such as postural dizziness/light-headedness, hypotension, or significant weight loss of greater than 1 kg sustained over one week, that may indicate the patient is hypovolaemic and requires a reduction in the dose of potassium losing diuretic (see Figure 9.5).

Digoxin

Digoxin should be considered for patients who, despite optimal doses of diuretics and ACE inhibitors, continue to have symptomatically severe heart failure, very poor left ventricular systolic function, or persisting cardiac dilation leading to recurrent hospital admissions. A number of studies have demonstrated that withdrawal of digoxin from patients with heart failure was associated with deteriorating heart failure symptoms and an increased risk of hospital admission. The DIG trial found that patients had a symptomatic improvement when digoxin was added to treatment with diuretics and ACE inhibitor therapy.[1,2,8]

Dose

The dose of digoxin should be aimed towards achieving a serum concentration within a therapeutic range of 0·6–2·6 nmol/l or 0·5–2·0 ng/ml. The median digoxin dose used in the PROVED Investigation Group and Randomized Assessment of Digoxin on Inhibitors of the Angiotensin Converting Enzyme (RADIANCE) trials

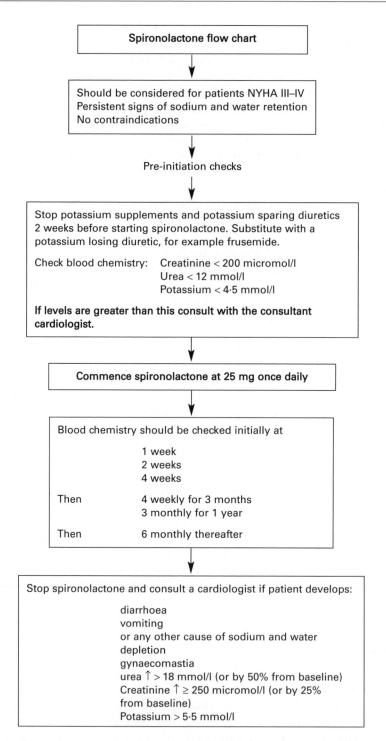

Figure 9.5 Guidance on spironolactone treatment in chronic heart failure

was approximately 0·375 mg.[1,2,8] In the Digitalis Intervention Group (DIG) trial the equivalent dose was 0·25 mg. In practice however it is not always possible to achieve these target doses unless the patient does not have a therapeutic serum concentration and their creatinine is less than 200 micromol/l and urea less than 15 micromol/l. In these cases the dose of digoxin can be increased by 0·0625 mg. Otherwise a maintenance dose of 0·125–0·375 mg should be given. A smaller dose may need to be considered for elderly patients whose renal function is impaired. Digoxin concentrations can also increase with drugs such as amiodarone and erythromycin, and therefore smaller doses may need to be used in these patients.

Key clinical issues

As digoxin toxicity can arise with any dose, it is important that the specialist nurse observes for signs of anorexia, nausea, vomiting, headache, xanthopsia (yellow tint to vision), bradycardia, and arrhythmias (for example atrial tachycardia, ventricular tachycardia, and atrio-ventricular blocks). Some patients, particularly the elderly, may manifest more subtle signs of confusion, reduced mobility, and falls that may be mistakenly identified as early dementia without monitoring of the serum digoxin concentration and appropriate adjustment of the dose.

Therapeutic monitoring

Close monitoring of blood chemistry is essential in patients receiving digoxin therapy as deteriorating renal function often leads to increases in digoxin concentrations leading to digoxin toxicity. The patient's physician/cardiologist should be alerted to serum creatinine levels > 200 micromol/l and urea level > 15 micromol/l. A digoxin level should be checked 14 days following the drug initiation or dosage alteration. In order to obtain a "trough" level, the assay is usually obtained six hours following their last dose. If the serum concentration is sub-therapeutic the patient's physician/cardiologist must be advised, the digoxin dose may be increased (by 0·0625 mg) and the same protocol used to monitor digoxin concentration will be applied. The physician/cardiologist should also be alerted if the serum concentration is above the therapeutic level, in which case the dose of digoxin will usually be reduced or in some instances hospital admission may be required to treat severe toxicity.

Angiotensin receptor blockers

Although the definitive role of this class of drugs in treating chronic heart failure is still to be determined following the recent results of the CHARM-Overall programme and pending update guidelines, there is little doubt its use will increase.[3-5] At present the strongest evidence supports the use of these agents (particularly candersartan) as an alternative to ACE inhibition in those intolerant of this class of agent.[4] There is also good evidence (once again from the CHARM-Added and CHARM-Preserved trials) that candersartan may be used in addition to ACE inhibition to improve clinical outcomes.[5,11]

Dose

The following represent the most commonly used angiotensin receptor blockers and their target doses (highest dose):

- losartan (12·5–50 mg once daily)
- candersartan (4–32 mg once daily)
- valsartan (40–160 mg once daily).

Figure 9.6 shows the titration regimen employed in the CHARM-Overall programme where physicians were able to decide whether to commence candersartan at either 4 or 8 mg once daily and increase the dosage every 14 days depending on the patient's underlying blood pressure and serum potassium and creatinine (see below): the major inference being that a lower dose be employed in those already receiving ACE inhibitor therapy and/or intolerant to ACE inhibition because of symptomatic blood pressure and/or renal dysfunction.

Key clinical issues

With the exception of a bradykinin related cough, these agents have a similar profile to ACE inhibitors. The same precautions apply – particularly when added to an ACE inhibitor (refer to the relevant ACE inhibitor section above).

Therapeutic monitoring

Once again, refer to the relevant ACE inhibitor section above.

Nitrates and hydralazine

Nitrates may still be used to treat persistent symptoms associated with chronic heart failure. If used in combination with hydralazine for patients already on a diuretic and/or digoxin they have been demonstrated to confer improvements in survival in patients with NYHA class II/III heart failure secondary to left ventricular systolic dysfunction.[1,2,8] Following recent studies, they are likely to be indicated for patients who are truly intolerant of ACE inhibitor and

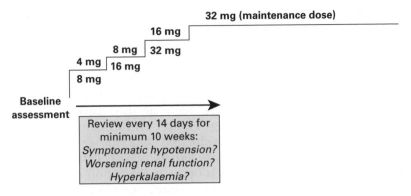

Figure 9.6 Up-titration of candersartan in chronic heart failure (irrespective of underlying left ventricular ejection fraction and concurrent ACE inhibitor therapy)

angiotensin receptor blocker therapy (approximately 20% of patients in the CHARM-Alternative study intolerant to ACE inhibition were also withdrawn from active therapy due to adverse events[5]).

Dose

Hydralazine is started at 37·5 mg four times a day and, if tolerated, increased 14 days later. The dose is then doubled until a maximum dose of 300 mg per day is reached. Isosorbide dinitrate is started at 20 mg four times a day and, if tolerated, is also increased 14 days later. The dose is then doubled until a maximum dose of 160 mg per day is reached. Smaller doses of each are considered for patients who are unable to tolerate the maximum dose.

Key clinical issues and therapeutic monitoring

Common problems associated with this treatment include dizziness, headaches, hypotension, gastric problems, tachycardia, palpitations, and fluid retention. All can be detected by regular follow-up and clinical assessment of the patient's weight, blood pressure, and heart rate, in particular prior to dosage increments.

Issues relating to non-chronic heart failure specific medications

A number of concomitant medications can aggravate chronic heart failure. These include non-steroidal anti-inflammatory drugs, larger doses of aspirin, and most calcium channel antagonists (the only likely exception being amlodipine). Lithium levels can be seriously affected by changes in diuretic doses. It is for this reason that patients on lithium will require medical supervision including liaison with the community psychiatric team.[8]

Many patients with arthritis may require treatment with a non-steroidal anti-inflammatory; this necessity should only be encouraged once alternative pain relief has been deemed ineffective. Non-steroidal anti-inflammatory drugs exhibit anti-inflammatory effects by inhibiting prostaglandin production (via the cyclo-oxygenase pathway). Prostaglandins in the kidney cause vasodilation and promote sodium excretion, which opposes the action of angiotensin II. Non-steroidal anti-inflammatory drugs therefore cause sodium retention and for this reason should be used cautiously in heart failure.[8]

The use of low dose aspirin as an antithrombotic agent is widespread in coronary artery disease. However subgroup analysis of ACE inhibitor trials in heart failure has shown that the benefit of these drugs was reduced in those patients taking aspirin. At present most opinion favours the continued use of aspirin in heart failure patients with coronary disease, to be taken in a dose of 75 mg daily.[8] The use of any calcium channel blocker should be questioned and if justified (usually only for angina) the only agent used should be amlodipine. Cardiology advice may be required.[8] Some over the counter and homeopathic preparations can interact with a number of cardiac medications. There is some evidence to suggest that St John's wort can interact with digoxin by reducing the digoxin level.

Treatment of gout in heart failure

Gout, a common condition in patients with chronic heart failure, is an acute arthritis that most commonly occurs in the first metatarsophalangeal joint (big toe) but can also affect other joints including the ankle and elbow, and in the hands. It often develops overnight and the patient wakes up with extreme pain in the morning.

Gout is caused by the deposition of monosodium urate crystals in the joint cavity. This occurs in the presence of high serum levels of uric acid (hyperuricaemia). Levels are usually > 600 micromol/l when gout occurs. However many patients tolerate this level without developing this condition. Uric acid is the end product of degradation of purines, which are an integral part of nucleic acids (DNA etc). Two thirds of uric acid is excreted via the kidneys and the remainder via the gut. Some consumables are also a high source of purines (for example beer).

Any condition that leads to high uric acid levels can cause gout. In heart failure, the commonest cause is the use of diuretics. All diuretics reduce the renal excretion of uric acid, although thiazides – such as bendrofluazide and metolazone – are particularly prone to do this. The loop diuretic torasemide may have less effect on uric acid levels. Low dose aspirin, commonly prescribed in heart disease, also impairs the excretion of uric acid. Alcohol raises uric acid levels by a number of mechanisms, and this may be an important cause in some patients. Other general causes include dieting or weight loss from any cause, and being male.

An acute episode of gout should be treated with a non-steroidal anti-inflammatory drug, such as indomethacin 50 mg three times per day, diclofenac (voltarol) 50 mg or naproxen 500 mg twice daily. This should be given for a short course of up to seven days to allow an attack to settle. Large prolonged doses should be avoided in heart failure because of the risks of fluid retention.[8] Other side effects include gastric irritation/ulcers and rashes.

If a non-steroidal anti-inflammatory drug appears to be absolutely contraindicated (for example in the presence of peptic ulcer disease) colchicine can be prescribed. This is given as a single dose of 1 mg, followed by 500 micrograms every 2–3 hours until an attack settles (maximum dose 10 mg, not repeated within three days). Colchicine is an antimitotic agent, which commonly causes abdominal pain, nausea, and diarrhoea.

After the acute attack has resolved, a decision may be taken to commence allopurinol. This drug inhibits xanthine oxidase, which is a key enzyme in the formation of uric acid. Allopurinol is usually not commenced unless more than one documented episode of gout has occurred. The initial dose is 100 mg once daily, which is increased over a few weeks to reduce uric acid levels to near the normal range. The usual maintenance dose is 300 mg daily. Allopurinol is generally well tolerated. Side effects include rash and gastric upset. Allopurinol should be commenced three weeks after an acute episode has resolved as starting it during an episode may prolong it indefinitely.

In patients with concurrent gout and heart failure, it is important to decide what is the most likely cause of raised uric acid levels. For example, it may be possible to reduce or alter the diuretic regimen, which may prevent further episodes of gout without the need for allopurinol.

Summary

Applying the evidence from clinical trials of pharmacological agents is not easy. Successful application of evidence-based therapies relies on a number of other contributory factors such as patient education, regular review, careful blood chemistry monitoring, patient compliance, good communication, and non-pharmacological

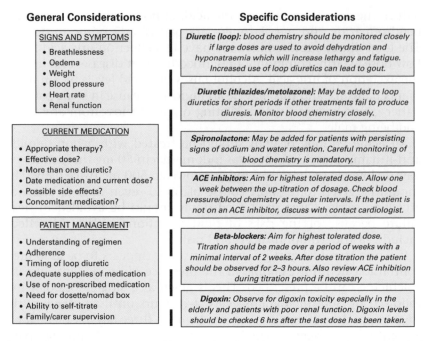

General Considerations	Specific Considerations
SIGNS AND SYMPTOMS • Breathlessness • Oedema • Weight • Blood pressure • Heart rate • Renal function	*Diuretic (loop): blood chemistry should be monitored closely if large doses are used to avoid dehydration and hyponatraemia which will increase lethargy and fatigue. Increased use of loop diuretics can lead to gout.*
	Diuretic (thiazides/metolazone): May be added to loop diuretics for short periods if other treatments fail to produce diuresis. Monitor blood chemistry closely.
CURRENT MEDICATION • Appropriate therapy? • Effective dose? • More than one diuretic? • Date medication and current dose? • Possible side effects? • Concomitant medication?	*Spironolactone: May be added for patients with persisting signs of sodium and water retention. Careful monitoring of blood chemistry is mandatory.*
	ACE inhibitors: Aim for highest tolerated dose. Allow one week between the up-titration of dosage. Check blood pressure/blood chemistry at regular intervals. If the patient is not on an ACE inhibitor, discuss with contact cardiologist.
PATIENT MANAGEMENT • Understanding of regimen • Adherence • Timing of loop diuretic • Adequate supplies of medication • Use of non-prescribed medication • Need for dosette/nomad box • Ability to self-titrate • Family/carer supervision	*Beta-blockers: Aim for highest tolerated dose. Titration should be made over a period of weeks with a minimal interval of 2 weeks. After dose titration the patient should be observed for 2–3 hours. Also review ACE inhibition during titration period if necessary*
	Digoxin: Observe for digoxin toxicity especially in the elderly and patients with poor renal function. Digoxin levels should be checked 6 hrs after the last dose has been taken.

Figure 9.7 General and specific considerations in managing a pharmacological regimen for chronic heart failure

intervention. Figure 9.7, in conjunction with the detailed description provided in previous chapters, outlines some of the important issues relating to the successful management of chronic heart failure using the most commonly used pharmacological agents.

References

1 Remme WJ, Swedberg K; Task Force for the Diagnosis and Treatment of Chronic Heart Failure, European Society of Cardiology. Guidelines for the diagnosis and treatment of chronic heart failure. *Eur Heart J* 2001;**22**:1527–60.

2 Hunt SA, Baker DW, Chin MH, *et al.* ACC/AHA Guidelines for the Evaluation and Management of Chronic Heart Failure in the Adult: Executive Summary. A Report of the American College of Cardiology/American Heart Association Task Force on Practice Guidelines (Committee to Revise the 1995 Guidelines for the Evaluation and Management of Heart Failure): Developed in Collaboration With the International Society for Heart and Lung Transplantation; Endorsed by the Heart Failure Society of America. *Circulation* 2001;**104**:2996–3007.

3 Pfeffer MA, Swedberg K, Granger CB, *et al.* Effects of candesartan on mortality and morbidity in patients with chronic heart failure: the CHARM-Overall programme. *Lancet* 2003;**362**:759–66.

4 McMurray JJ, Ostergren J, Swedberg K, *et al.* Effects of candesartan in patients with chronic heart failure and reduced left ventricular systolic function taking angiotensin-converting-enzyme inhibitors: the CHARM-Added Trial. *Lancet* 2003;**362**:767–71.

5   Granger CB, McMurray JJV, Yusuf S, *et al.* Effects of candesartan in patients with chronic heart failure and reduced left-ventricular systolic function intolerant to angiotensin-converting-enzyme inhibitors: the CHARM-Alternative Trial. *Lancet* 2003;**362**:772–6.

6   Petrie MC, Berry C, Stewart S, McMurray JJ. Failing ageing hearts. *Eur Heart J* 2001;**22**:1978–90.

7   Masoudi FA, Havranek EP, Wolfe P, *et al.* Most hospitalized older persons do not meet the enrollment criteria for clinical trials in heart failure. *Am Heart J* 2003;**146**:250–7.

8   McMurray J, Cohen-Solal A, Dietz R, *et al.* Practical recommendations for the use of ACE inhibitors, beta-blockers and spironolactone in heart failure: putting guidelines into practice. *Eur J Heart Fail* 2001;**3**:495–502.

9   MacIntyre K, Capewell S, Stewart S, *et al.* Evidence of improving prognosis in heart failure: trends in case fatality in 66 547 patients hospitalized between 1986 and 1995. *Circulation* 2000;**102**:1126–31.

10 Wolny A, Clozel JP, Rein J, *et al.* Functional and biochemical analysis of angiotensin II-forming pathways in the human heart. *Circ Res* 1997;**80**:219–27.

11 Yusuf S, Pfeffer MA, Swedberg K, *et al.* Effects of candesartan in patients with chronic heart failure and preserved left-ventricular ejection fraction: the CHARM-Preserved Trial. *Lancet* 2003;**362**:777–81.

Section 4:
The future

10: New frontiers in specialist nurse management of heart failure

LYNDA BLUE, SIMON STEWART

Introduction

In these past few years it has become increasingly evident that heart failure as a truly malignant, debilitating, and costly syndrome has finally attracted the kind of attention and resources it deserves.[1,2] One only has to examine the increasing size, vibrancy, and diversity of research presented at the annual scientific meetings of the Heart Failure Society of America and the Heart Failure Working Group for the European Society of Cardiology to gauge the high degree of attention now directed towards solving the problems inherent to an epidemic of heart failure.

With this attention has come an increasing awareness that without a legitimate and widely available cure our best efforts merely prolong an inevitable but often unpredictable decline in the functional status and quality of life of patients with this syndrome.[3] It is within this essentially grim context that the evidence for applying predominantly nurse-led programmes of care, designed to optimise the management of those who have been hospitalised with chronic heart failure, has been strengthened considerably.[4,5] The past 3–5 years have seen a dramatic rise in the number of academics and clinicians convinced by the need for widespread application of specific programmes of heart failure care, in order to cost-effectively reduce recurrent readmissions, improve quality of life and perhaps prolong survival in typically older patients in whom treatment options are limited and/or difficult to apply. Meta-analyses of randomised studies certainly provide compelling evidence to support this view.[6,7]

This "good news" has to be tempered, however, with the realisation that some things have not changed. For example, without a cure, the prevalence of heart failure continues to rise and predictions of a sustained epidemic in the 21st century are still well founded with little relief in sight.[8,9] Given the ongoing individual and societal burden imposed by heart failure, therefore, it is disappointing to note that the types of programme described in our first edition are still not applied as widely as they should be. This is despite the wealth of evidence, and its incorporation into expert heart failure treatment guidelines. Part of the problem is undoubtedly cost considerations within financially stressed healthcare systems. Another problem is a lack of appreciation of the depth of evidence from a wide range of countries to support their application among healthcare administrators. Finally and most importantly, there is the common problem of "good intent" and funding to apply heart failure programmes but without specific blueprints and expertise to actually implement the evidence in a cost-effective manner.

Fortunately, the pool of expertise and material relating to the cost-effectiveness of nurse-led heart failure management is slowly increasing on an international basis. As such there are a number of factors that will *probably* ensure that the rising number of practising specialist heart failure nurses do not suddenly find themselves unemployed in the next five years or so. Four of the most important of these factors are as follows.

- The progressive ageing of the population,[10] combined with improved survival rates from previously fatal cardiac events associated with underlying and incurable heart disease,[11] will produce an inexorable rise in the prevalence of heart failure[8,9] – even if, as discussed in Chapter 1, the incidence of heart failure falls.[11]
- Heart failure is an international phenomenon. With increased access to the world wide web and widely distributed international expert guidelines[12,13] it is difficult for any one healthcare system and its administrators to continually avoid the compelling evidence of a heart failure epidemic, and the value of specialist heart failure nurses to combat it. Certainly, consumers affected by heart failure are unlikely to accept being deprived of such potent "treatment".
- The cost dynamics of the heart failure burden, with healthcare expenditure predominantly attributable to hospitalisation, combined with the attractiveness of programmes that alter the pattern of health care to more cost-effective community based management, provides a compelling economic argument for employing specialist heart failure nurses (see Chapter 5).
- There is widespread recognition that the impressive results from clinical trials of new pharmacological agents in heart failure (for example CHARM,[14] COPERNICUS,[15] MERIT,[16] CIBIS II,[17] and RALES[18]) will never be translated into the "real world" without specialist heart failure nurses to implement new therapies in already complex treatment regimens.

Until an effective (and cheap) cure for hypertension, coronary heart disease, and/or heart failure is found, therefore, the need for the type of programme outlined in this book will be sustained.

New frontiers for specialist heart failure nurses

Assuming that specialist heart failure nurses will be a valuable, cost-effective and more common feature of healthcare systems over the next five to ten years, what are the clinical issues and developments that are likely to provide new opportunities to improve the post-discharge management of patients with heart failure and also expand the role of the specialist nurse beyond current boundaries?

Improving current practice

Before discussing some of the key developments likely to improve the effectiveness of nurse-led management programmes in heart failure, it is important to note that aiming for an almost complete obliteration of hospital episodes relating to heart failure and those conditions closely linked to such morbidity is unrealistic. The same applies to preventing heart failure related mortality. It is clear, however, that there is much more to achieve in relation to improving health outcomes in heart failure with the important aim of minimising emergency hospital admissions, prolonging life, and improving quality of life. The following represent emerging therapeutic strategies that are likely to become fully integrated into heart failure management programmes to achieve these aims in the near future.

Interactive monitoring of patients in their own home

As discussed in more detail in Chapter 3, there is growing interest in the role of interactive technology to provide greater surveillance and follow-up of patients with chronic heart failure. For example, the recently reported Trans European Network Homecare Monitoring Study (TEN-HMS)[19] involving 427 patients, a third of whom were randomised to a telemonitoring protocol, when published in its full form will stimulate much debate as to the utility of such technology. As such, while there have been attempts to replace personal contact in the form of clinic and home visits with different forms of telephonic and interactive follow-up in heart failure[20-23] it would appear likely that such technology would be used in an adjunctive capacity to support current forms of management in the future. There is a strong case, however, for using such technology (once it has been proven to be user-friendly and cost-effective) to monitor patients who are distant from personal, expert cardiac care (for example outback Australia).

Monitoring brain natriuretic peptide concentrations to optimise therapy

As discussed in Chapter 3, there is increasing evidence to suggest that serial monitoring of B-type natriuretic peptide (BNP) and N-terminal pro-BNP (NT-BNP) BNP and NT-BNP concentrations in the blood of patients being aggressively treated for chronic heart failure is likely to improve health outcomes. Concentrations of these peptides correlate with the haemodynamic profile and clinical severity of underlying heart failure. Importantly, higher BNP or NT-BNP value indicates a greater risk of hospitalisation or death.[24-29] Following reports that patients with the lowest BNP concentrations have the best clinical outcomes,[30,31] a recent pilot study undertaken by a New Zealand team demonstrated that tailoring management of chronic heart failure to actively lower the production of these potent peptides led to better health outcomes.[24]

At present there are a number of large-scale studies (including one involving the Glasgow Heart Failure Liaison Service) examining whether actively monitoring BNP levels in chronic heart failure is a cost-effective strategy to further reduce morbidity and prolong survival. In all likelihood, such studies will lead to the introduction of this type of monitoring – particularly if the cost of measurement is reduced and "point-of-care" results are available to make rapid clinical decisions.[32]

Extending current practice

There are two major areas of clinical practice, at the opposite ends of the clinical spectrum encompassing heart failure, that offer the most promise in terms of extending the role of the specialist heart failure nurse. Both have the potential to deliver significant benefits to the community. These comprise the early detection and management of "latent" heart failure in the community and the care of patients with end-stage heart failure to provide quality end of life.

Early detection and management of heart failure in the community

As described in Chapter 1, the number of individuals within the population with "latent" heart failure is likely to be equally as great as those who have already developed the classic signs and symptoms usually associated with the syndrome of heart failure. It is within this context that the recent update of the AHA/ACC guidelines for the management of heart failure also needs to be considered.[13] In response to the evolving epidemiologic profile of cardiovascular disease, this expert committee proposed a new way of tackling an epidemic of heart failure. In a new classification system, they identified four stages of heart failure with the following relevant features:

Stage A Individuals at high risk of developing heart failure: those with pre-existing hypertension, coronary artery disease, left bundle branch block, diabetes, and/or a body mass index of > 30 kg/m^2 (obesity)

Stage B Individuals with previous AMI, asymptomatic valvular disease, and/or asymptomatic left ventricular systolic dysfunction

Stage C Individuals with symptomatic heart failure

Stage D Patients with severe chronic heart failure who have been admitted to hospital.[13]

Not unexpectedly, much attention has been paid to those who can be classified as Stage D (hence this book). Much less attention has been paid to optimising the detection and management of Stage A patients who spend the majority of their time in the community and are predominantly managed by primary care physicians/general practitioners. Those who would be considered to be in Stage A and at high risk of developing heart failure without appropriate attention represent a particularly neglected patient cohort. As such, with a high prevalence of individuals with co-factors other than ischaemic heart disease that will almost inevitably lead to the development of overt heart failure (for example hypertension[33] and obesity[34]) there is an urgent need to now focus on the detection and management of patients in AHA/ACC/ESC Stages A, B, and C.

As noted, these patients are most likely to be managed within the primary healthcare sector. Given limited resources and, to date, difficulty in determining the potential presence of heart failure, they more than likely receive sub-optimal treatment to prevent further progression to more severe heart failure. As such, there is a growing debate in respect to the provision of cost-effective and large-scale screening programmes for patients with a history suggestive of heart failure that present to their general practitioner. The most likely candidate for patient screening involves the measurement of BNP concentrations with the combination of a higher concentration and an abnormal ECG in "high risk" patients (for example aged > 55 years and with one or more risk factors for heart disease) prompting further, more definitive, investigation (for example echocardiography) and treatment of underlying heart failure/left ventricular systolic dysfunction if detected.[35]

Any programme of this type needs to be pragmatic and use pre-existing resources in a cost-effective way. Given the increasing pressure on general practitioner workloads, practice nurses represent a potentially important vehicle to screen for patients at risk of developing heart failure (Stage A) and addressing modifiable risk factors. Furthermore, they could detect patients who have already developed the syndrome of heart failure (Stages B and C) in order to facilitate a definitive diagnosis (i.e. preserved or systolic dysfunction) and management according to current guidelines.[13]

If current trials do show such screening programmes are effective, where does the specialist heart failure nurse fit in? Clearly, with increased detection of patients with heart failure and the consequent need to provide them with effective therapy the expertise of the specialist nurse will be invaluable – particularly if they are able to facilitate and guide practice nurses and general practitioners in their primary role for detection and management. This assumes that the specialist nurse would act in a supportive role rather than assume total control – a common fear among those who operate within primary care. As such, this role would formalise what many specialist nurses already do – act as a valuable resource to support the primary care management of heart failure, regardless of whether affected patients are enrolled in their service or not.

Palliative care in heart failure

The advanced stages of heart failure can have a devastating effect on a patient's quality of life. At present, patients with chronic heart failure and their carers have limited access to palliative care. Much has been done for patients with cancer, but the needs of those with chronic heart failure have been neglected,[36] Reasons for the absence of palliative care services include a lack of resources and expertise, and problems associated with determining prognosis. Most of the usually elderly patients with heart failure have short lives of extremely poor quality, punctuated by frequent admissions to hospital.[37,38]

Research by Hanratty and colleagues[39] to determine the views of general practitioners and specialists in cardiology, geriatric medicine, and palliative medicine in the north of England found the overall picture was grim, describing poor quality of care for patients and frustration amongst doctors. They also noted that predicting the illness trajectory in end stage heart failure patients is much harder when compared to those with terminal malignancy. This creates uncertainty and can potentially prevent doctors telling patients when they have reached the terminal phase of their illness and planning appropriate care.

Murray and colleagues[40] described the experiences and views of patients dying from heart failure or lung cancer. They also interviewed their carers (see Appendix 3). As identified in the study by Hanratty, the illness trajectory of lung cancer was much more predictable than for heart failure. Participants reported poor coordination and inadequate continuity of care with a single health care professional. Ward states there is a need for research into the use and action of opioids in chronic heart failure, which should include the evaluation of different treatment regimens, and the use of alternative opioid delivery systems.[41] A pilot study on the use of morphine for the relief of breathlessness in patients with chronic heart failure by Johnson and colleagues reported that "oral morphine gave clinically significant improvement in breathlessness to those patients with advanced heart failure".[42]

It seems obvious that further research and resources are required to develop appropriate models of care to meet the specific needs of patients with chronic heart failure. But who can provide this additional care in a cost-effective manner? Fortunately, specialist heart failure nurses already possess most of the required skills and are becoming proactive participants in the process of providing quality end of life care in heart failure by firstly addressing a key issue.

How many patients specifically require palliative care? The number of patients requiring palliative care for end stage heart failure is relatively small but their management is labour intensive and complex. In the Glasgow Heart Failure Liaison Service for example we estimate approximately 60 patients per year will require end of life care. Many patients have one or more clinically important comorbidities (e.g. renal and respiratory dysfunction) that often complicate their management and add to the burden imposed by chronic refractory symptoms. Having identified the likely scope of the problem, there are a number of important related issues that need to be addressed.

Identifying the right patients for palliative care These patients have frequent recurrent hospital admissions with symptoms indicative of NYHA Class IV refractory to maximal therapy. They often exhibit worsening oedema and experience progressive renal failure before dying. There appear to be a number of key elements required to identify the patient who has severe chronic heart failure refractory to medical (or surgical) treatment. These include:

- availability of protocols for the management of refractory heart failure ensuring that a reversible aetiology or precipitant has not been overlooked and that all reasonable treatment options have been considered – this will enable healthcare professionals to identify the terminal stage of heart failure and its management

- identifying what is appropriate management (i.e. symptom relief, diuretics, pain control)
- identifying what is inappropriate management (i.e. inotropes, dialysis, central lines, and urinary catheters – unless the patient has a retention or for his/her comfort, not just to monitor urinary output)
- good coordination and continuity of care by a single healthcare professional to determine whether the patient experiences periodic episodes of severe heart failure due to other extraneous factors (for example non-adherence to treatment) or simply as part of the natural history of their particular form of heart failure.

Key components of palliative care in heart failure   Likewise, the application of an effective management plan to ease the suffering associated with end stage heart failure has to involve a number of key elements.

- A formal case conference involving all members of the patient's multidisciplinary management team to develop a palliative care plan. The number of health and social care professionals involved will vary from one area to another. However, it is vital that all key members of the team are involved in the decision making process.
- A mechanism to communicate and document the patient's management to relevant health and social care professionals following hospital discharge ensuring clarity about what the management plan is.
- If the patient is discharged to their home an adequate package of care has to be implemented.
- If the patient is discharged to hospice care communication links must be established with heart failure expertise to support nursing and medical staff in managing the patient's care.
- Ensuring that an updated management plan is included in the patient's general practice and hospital case notes. For example, if a decision is made to avoid active resuscitation in the event of cardiorespiratory arrest, all clinicians should be made aware of this fact.

Regular clinical review

This is certainly an evolving and important field of endeavour for specialist heart failure nurses and one that will require close attention and planning in future years. Hopefully, protocols and formal support services to implement best practice in palliative care management in heart failure will be available in the near future.

Summary

The need for heart failure services in which the specialist heart failure nurse plays a central role has never been stronger. Given the likelihood of a sustained epidemic of this debilitating syndrome,[8,9] the implications of studies such as CHARM[14] and that undertaken by Moser and colleagues[43] that suggest we can do more for patients with preserved systolic function (otherwise known as diastolic heart failure), and the prospect of greater involvement in early management as well as palliative care for heart failure, the role of the specialist heart failure nurse will evolve and expand for the foreseeable future.

References

1   Parmley WW. Heart failure awareness week: February 14–21. *J Am Coll Cardiol* 2000;**35**:534.
2   Konstam MA. Progress in heart failure management? Lessons from the real world. *Circulation* 2000;**102**:1076–8.
3   Stewart S, McMurray JJ. Palliative care for heart failure? *BMJ* 2002;**325**:915–6.
4   Stewart S, Horowitz JD. Specialist nurse management programmes: economic benefits in the management of heart failure. *Pharmacoeconomics* 2003;**21**:225–40.
5   Rich MW. Heart failure disease management: a critical review. *J Cardiac Fail* 1999; **5**:64–75.
6   McAlister FA, Lawson FM, Teo KK, Armstrong PW. A systematic review of randomized trials of disease management programs in heart failure. *Am J Med* 2001;**110**:378–84.
7   Stewart S, Berry C, McMurray JJV. Multidisciplinary intervention in congestive heart failure – does it reduce morbidity and mortality? *Eur Heart J* 2003;**24**:65.
8   Bonneux L, Barendregt JJ, Meeter K, Bonsel GJ, van der Maas PJ. Estimating clinical morbidity due to ischemic heart disease and congestive heart failure: the future rise of heart failure. *Am J Public Health* 1994;**84**:20–8.
9   Stewart S, MacIntyre K, Capewell S, McMurray JJ. Heart failure and the aging population: an increasing burden in the 21st Century? *Heart* 2003;**89**:49–53.
10 Lindbloom E. America's aging population: changing the face of health care. *JAMA* 1993;**269**:674, 679.
11 Hellermann JP, Goraya TY, Jacobsen SJ, *et al*. Incidence of heart failure after myocardial infarction: is it changing over time? *Am J Epidemiol* 2003;**157**:1101–7.
12 Remme WJ, Swedberg K. Guidelines for the diagnosis and treatment of chronic heart failure. *Eur Heart J* 2001;**22**:1527–60.
13 Hunt SA, Baker OW, Chin MH, *et al*. ACC/AHA Guidelines for the Evaluation and Management of Chronic Heart Failure in the Adult: Executive Summary. A Report of the American College of Cardiology/American Heart Association Task Force on Practice Guidelines (Committee to Revise the 1995 Guidelines for the Evaluation and Management of Heart Failure): Developed in Collaboration With the International Society for Heart and Lung Transplantation; Endorsed by the Heart Failure Society of America. *Circulation* 2001;**104**:2996–3007.
14 Pfeffer MA, Swedberg K, Granger CB, *et al*. Effects of candesartan on mortality and morbidity in patients with chronic heart failure: the CHARM-Overall programme. *Lancet* 2003;**362**:59–66.
15 Packer M, Coats AJ, Fowler MB, *et al*. for the Carvedilol Prospective Randomised Cumulative Survival Study Group. Effect of carvedilol on survival in severe chronic heart failure. *N Engl J Med* 2001;**344**:1651–8.
16 MERIT Investigators. Effect of metoprolol CR/XL in chronic heart failure: Metoprolol CR/XL Randomised Intervention Trial in Congestive Heart Failure (Merit-HF). *Lancet* 1999;**353**:2001–7.

17 CIBIS-II Investigators and Committees. The Cardiac Insufficiency Bisoprolol Study II (CIBIS-II): a randomised trial. *Lancet* 1999;**353**:9–13.

18 Pitt B, Zannad F, Remme WJ, *et al*. The effect of spironolactone on morbidity and mortality in patients with severe heart failure. Randomized Aldactone Evaluation Study Investigators. *N Engl J Med* 1999;**341**:709–17.

19 Coletta AP, Louis AA, Clark AL, *et al*. Clinical trials update from the European Society of Cardiology: CARMEN, EARTH, OPTIMAAL, ACE, TEN-HMS, MAGIC, SOLVD-X and PATH-CHF II. *Eur J Heart Fail* 2002;**4**:661–6.

20 Riegel B, Carlson B, Kopp Z, LePetri B, Glaser D, Unger A. Effect of a standardized nurse case-management telephone intervention on resource use in patients with chronic heart failure. *Arch Intern Med* 2002;**162**:705–12.

21 Jerant AF, Azari R, Nesbitt TS. Reducing the cost of frequent hospital admissions for congestive heart failure: a randomized trial of a home telecare intervention. *Med Care* 2001;**39**:1234–45.

22 Shah NB, Der E, Ruggerio C, Heidenreich PA, Massie BM. Prevention of hospitalizations for heart failure with an interactive home monitoring program. *Am Heart J* 1998;**135**:373–8.

23 de Lusignan S, Wells S, Johnson P, Meredith K, Leatham E. Compliance and effectiveness of 1 year's home telemonitoring. The report of a pilot study of patients with chronic heart failure. *Eur J Heart Fail* 2001;**3**:723–30.

24 Troughton RW, Frampton CM, Yandle TG, Espiner EA, Frampton CM, Nicholls MG, Richards AM. Treatment of heart failure guided by plasma aminoterminal brain natriuretic peptide (N-BNP) concentrations. *Lancet* 2000;**355**:1126–30.

25 Berger R, Stanek B, Frey B, *et al*. B-type natriuretic peptides (BNP and PRO-BNP) predict longterm survival in patients with advanced heart failure treated with atenolol. *J Heart Lung Transplant* 2001; **20**:251.

26 McDonagh TA, Cunningham AD, Morrison CE, *et al*. Left ventricular dysfunction, natriuretic peptides, and mortality in an urban population. *Heart* 2001;**86**:21–6.

27 Berger R, Huelsman M, Strecker K, *et al*. B-type natriuretic peptide predicts sudden death in patients with chronic heart failure. *Circulation* 2002;**105**:2392–7.

28 Anand IS, Fisher LD, Chiang YT, *et al*. Changes in brain natriuretic peptide and norepinephrine over time and mortality and morbidity in the Valsartan Heart Failure Trial (Val-HeFT). *Circulation* 2003;**107**:1278–83.

29 Fisher C, Berry C, Blue L, Morton J, McMurray JJ. N-terminal pro B type natriuretic peptide, but not the new putative cardiac hormone relaxin, predicts prognosis in patients with chronic heart failure. *Heart* 2003;**89**:879–81.

30 Cheng V, Kazanagra R, Garcia A, *et al*. A rapid bedside test for B-type peptide predicts treatment outcomes in patients admitted for decompensated heart failure: a pilot study. *J Am Coll Cardiol* 2001;**37**:386–91.

31 Bettencourt P, Ferreira S, Azevedo A, Ferreira A. Preliminary data on the potential usefulness of B-type natriuretic peptide levels in predicting outcome after hospital discharge in patients with heart failure. *Am J Med* 2002;**113**:215–9.

32 Safley DM, McCullough PA. The emerging role of brain natriuretic peptide in the management of acute and chronic heart failure in outpatients. *Heart Fail Monit* 2003; **4**:13–20.

33 Chobanian AV, Bakris GL, Black HR, *et al*. for the National Heart, Lung, and Blood Institute Joint National Committee on Prevention, Detection, Evaluation, and Treatment of High Blood Pressure; National High Blood Pressure Education Program Coordinating Committee. The Seventh Report of the Joint National Committee on Prevention, Detection, Evaluation, and Treatment of High Blood Pressure: the JNC 7 report. *JAMA* 2003;**289**(19):2560–72.

34 Kenchaiah S, Evans JC, Levy D, *et al*. Obesity and the risk of heart failure. *N Engl J Med* 2002;**347**:305–13.

35 Nielsen OW, McDonagh TA, Robb SD, Dargie HJ. Retrospective analysis of the cost-effectiveness of using plasma brain natriuretic peptide in screening for left ventricular systolic dysfunction in the general population. *J Am Coll Cardiol* 2003; **41**:113–20.

36 Jones S. Palliative care in terminal cardiac failure [Letter]. *BMJ* 1995;**310**:805.

37 Juenger J, Schellberg D, Kraemer S, *et al*. Health related quality of life in patients with congestive heart failure: comparison with other chronic diseases and relation to functional variables. *Heart* 2002;**87**:235–41.

38 Cowie MR, Fox KF, Wood DA, *et al.* Hospitalization of patients with heart failure: a population-based study. *Eur Heart J* 2002;**23**:877–85.

39 Hanratty B, Hibbert D, Mair F, *et al.* Doctors' perceptions of palliative care for heart failure: focus study group. *BMJ* 2002;**325**:581–5.

40 Murray SA, Boyd K, Kendall M, Worth A, Benton TF, Clausen H. Dying of lung cancer or cardiac failure: prospective qualitative interview study of patients and their carers in the community. *BMJ* 2002;**325**:929.

41 Ward C. The need for Palliative Care in the management of heart failure. *Heart* 2002;**87**:294–8.

42 Johnson M, McDonagh TA, Harkness A, McKay SE, Dargie HJ. Morphine for the relief of breathlessness in patients with chronic heart failure – a pilot study. *Eur J Heart Fail* 2002;**4**:753–6.

43 Moser DK, Macko MJ, Worster P. Community case management decreases rehospitalisation rates and costs, and improves quality of life in heart failure patients with preserved and non-preserved left ventricular function: a randomized controlled trial. *Circulation* 2000;**102**:II 749.

Appendices: some practical advice

Appendix 1: Profile of the specialist heart failure nurse: qualifications and training

LYNDA BLUE

Appointing and training personnel

One of the key components in successfully managing patients with chronic heart failure is the experience and expertise of the specialist nurse. Without the appointment of nurses who are highly motivated, and who have demonstrated expertise in the management of heart failure and the ability to use their own initiative, there is a high probability that the service will fail to reach its full potential. In order to select the right personnel, it is important to attract quality candidates by offering a generous salary package and the opportunity to perform in an innovative and rewarding role, and then to apply a rigorous selection process.

Essential qualifications

Potential candidates for the position of specialist nurse in heart failure should fit the following profile:

- professional nursing qualification (for example Registered Nurse with at least five years' experience)
- at least two years' recent cardiology experience
- community experience desirable (especially if home based intervention)
- excellent communication skills
- experience of working in an autonomous position
- a proven ability to work effectively in a multidisciplinary setting
- computing skills advantageous
- driving licence if community based.

Additional qualifications

When interviewing potential candidates, the following attributes should be used to assess the candidates on a more definitive basis:

- previous community based nursing experience
- specific expertise in managing patients with heart failure
- post-basic qualifications (for example, Critical Care Certificate) and/or higher nursing qualifications (BSc/Masters level)
- experience in research and/or auditing
- advanced information technology skills.

Training programme

Regardless of their expertise and qualifications, it is vital that all newly appointed specialist nurses undertake a comprehensive training programme prior to assuming responsibility for the recruitment and management of patients. In the Glasgow Heart Failure Liaison Service, for example, all appointed specialist heart failure nurses undertake a four-week induction programme.

The training programme should incorporate a large component of practical exposure to the day to day roles of the various healthcare professionals who are commonly involved in the management of patients with heart failure – both in the hospital and in community settings (for example hospital based staff, general practitioner/primary care physician, pharmacist, district nurse, practice nurse, and dietician). It is also valuable if the newly appointed nurses are able to accompany experienced healthcare professionals at a heart failure clinic and/or on visits to patients' homes.

A programme of heart failure management should be based on the recognition that all professionals managing patients with heart failure should:

- have the appropriate knowledge and skills to comprehensively assess and meet the individual needs of the patient in their care
- have access to a multidisciplinary team and utilise this appropriately to meet the individual patient's needs
- be informed by research and current evidence
- utilise objective outcome measures to determine effectiveness of treatment
- promote awareness of heart failure assessment, diagnosis, treatment and its effectiveness amongst other healthcare professionals.

Example of programme content

- Epidemiology/prognosis in heart failure
- Anatomy, physiology and pathophysiology of CHF
- Investigations and diagnosis/role of BNP/echocardiography
- Clinical assessment/examination/history taking/signs and symptoms
- Pharmacology
- Update of clinical trials – current gold standard pharmacological treatment of heart failure and applying medical guidelines to optimise such treatment
- Practical aspects of pharmacological management
- Optimising day to day management/improving adherence/non-pharmacological strategies
- Managing CHF patients with comorbidities
- Managing patients with progressive symptoms/palliative support/end of life care
- Exercise/rehabilitation
- Nutrition and cachexia
- Anaemia in heart failure
- Managing atrial fibrillation in patients with CHF
- Managing CHF patients with impaired renal function
- Changing technologies and the impact on patient management
- Quality of life/supporting patients and their carers, chronic illness and the impact on family and their carers
- Role of clinical psychologist in supporting patients with chronic conditions/CHF
- Patient information, education, and benefits
- Bridging the primary/secondary care interface
- Audit and evaluation
- Public health issues/cost of care – how the various components of health-care systems are linked at an operational level, role and cost of both hospital based health care and community based health care
- Coordinating health care, referring patients to other health care professionals
- Medicolegal issues/communication/documentation/record keeping/security
- Professional development
- Independent prescribing/supplementary prescribing
- Cultural issues
- Interdisciplinary perspectives
- Setting up service, models of care
- Case studies

Appendix 2: Case studies in managing chronic heart failure

Introduction

The following case studies represent a broad range of patients managed by specialist heart failure nurses and the often difficult issues that arise when attempting to improve each patient's quality of life and minimise their prospects of hospital readmission and a premature death. These case studies have been selected and presented by specialist heart failure nurses actively managing patients within the Glasgow Heart Failure Liaison Service. Although these case studies are based on real individuals, the demographic details of each have been altered to protect their anonymity.

Each case study has been written on an individual basis. As such, each author has highlighted the aspects of their case that they believe are most instructive and represent issues that cause the most difficulty when optimising the post-discharge management of a diverse range of patients with chronic heart failure.

Case study 1: Optimising pharmacotherapy in a 52-year-old woman with a diagnosis of cardiomyopathy following chemotherapy

KATRIONA MULLEN

Clinical background

This case study concerns a 52-year-old woman (Mrs A) with a brief but extremely unfortunate clinical history leading to the development of chronic heart failure. In 1998 Mrs A underwent a mastectomy to remove a breast tumour. In 2001 she developed auxiliary node recurrence with subsequent surgical removal of these nodes followed by treatment with the cytotoxic drug adriamycin.

Six months later she was readmitted to hospital with dyspnoea, extreme fatigue, paroxysmal nocturnal dyspnoea, and peripheral oedema extending to her sacrum. Chest radiograph showed interstitial oedema and cardiomegaly. Echocardiography revealed moderate to severe left ventricular systolic dysfunction. Mrs A was diagnosed with cardiomyopathy caused by administration of the cytotoxic drug adriamycin.

First home visit

I first visited Mrs A five days after hospital discharge. She lives with her family and has a reasonable level of social and practical support. At this first assessment she reported feeling relatively well and described a level of activity surprising considering her ventricular function. The following are the key features of my assessment of her condition at this time.

- She could walk a good distance on the flat (550 m), only becoming dyspnoeic when walking uphill. I assessed her as being NYHA Class II.
- She had no peripheral oedema and was managing to sleep soundly at night using two pillows.
- Blood pressure was 90/55 mmHg and pulse was 80 bpm regular. As such, she was hypotensive but asymptomatic. There was no postural difference in blood pressure.
- Blood screens showed near normal renal function with a urea of 6·2 mmol/l, creatinine of 61 micromol/l and potassium of 3·9 mmol/l.
- Liver function was abnormal: alkaline phosphatase 484 U/l and gamma GT of 260 micromol/l.
- Total cholesterol was high at 7·2 mmol/l.

Prescribed pharmacotherapy

- captopril 6·25 mg three times daily
- bisoprolol 1·25 mg daily
- furosemide 80 mg morning and 40 mg in the afternoon
- spironolactone 25 mg daily.

Patient education started at this first visit beginning with the priority of medication adherence. I checked Mrs A's hospital supply of tablets to assess adherence and discussed the actions of each drug with her. She had organised her new prescription with her general practitioner. I advised her to visit the same pharmacy each time she required more medication and emphasised that this is extremely useful when up-titrating any heart failure medication. I explained that the pharmacist becomes familiar with the client and their medication regimen and readily appreciates the need to frequently alter medication dosages according to the client's changing symptoms and optimisation of therapy.

I provided Mrs A with information about her heart failure, with particular reference to the underlying pathology and reasons for the symptoms she had experienced. In order to monitor Mrs A's condition I asked her to check and record her weight on a daily basis.

Next to medication adherence, I believe the issue of when to seek help and assistance is the next priority in patient education. I therefore gave Mrs A my contact phone number and encouraged her to contact me should she have any changing symptoms or sustained weight gain.

Initial management plan

Following this first assessment, my initial priority was to up-titrate the prescribed dose of both captopril and bisoprolol. I noted Mrs A's hypotension and reviewed her hospital records which showed this was a persistent problem. I decided to start with the captopril and increase the night-time dose to 12·5 mg, believing this was the safest option. Mrs A's liver function had been abnormal since her initial chemotherapy treatment. She had a liver ultrasound scan which showed no abnormalities, but I planned to continue monitoring her liver function. Mrs A's total cholesterol was also high. Since she had no ischaemic aetiology to her heart failure, I provided dietary advice and decided to check a fasting sample on a future visit because, considering her abnormal liver function test, it may not have been appropriate for Mrs A to be prescribed a statin.

Subsequent management

I reviewed Mrs A's condition within one week to assess her response to the increased captopril dose and continue with the educational process. At this time her blood pressure had fallen to 85/50 mmHg. However, she remained asymptomatic. Her urea concentration had increased to 9·2 mmol/l with no significant rise in creatinine. Her weight had not altered over the course of the week. She had no increase in her level of dyspnoea and no signs of fluid retention. In response I reduced the dose of furosemide to 80 mg daily.

I assessed her response to this medication change again within one week. Her urea concentration had reduced to 6·9 mmol/l and blood pressure had increased to 105/55 mmHg. Her weight had been static over the week. When spironolactone is used as well as a loop diuretic, the combination can sometimes allow for a reduction in the dose of loop diuretic as occurred in this case.

Over the course of the next month I increased both the morning and afternoon dose of captopril to 12·5 mg at two weekly intervals (dose now 12·5 mg three times daily). Renal function remained stable and systolic blood pressure ranged between 90 and 100 mmHg.

Symptomatically, Mrs A remained stable in NYHA Class II until she decided to take a holiday abroad with her family. Prior to her holiday I advised Mrs A to ensure an adequate fluid intake in the hot climate she was travelling to and to seek prompt medical advice should she suffer any prolonged vomiting or diarrhoea – both important points to emphasise in relation to her prescribed spironolactone. Mrs A remained well whilst abroad. However, on her return home she contacted me to report some worsening symptoms. She was dyspnoeic moving around her home and had some ankle oedema. Her weight had increased by 2 kg. Mrs A's blood pressure was now 85/50 mmHg. She also had a cough that was productive and her sputum was discoloured. I therefore contacted her general practitioner who prescribed a broad-spectrum antibiotic for an underlying chest infection. Any chest infection requires prompt treatment as there may be associated decompensation due to increased pulmonary resistance. I increased Mrs A's dose of furosemide by 40 mg. Within three days Mrs A felt some improvement in terms of her symptoms. Her weight had reduced by 1·5 kg and the ankle oedema had lessened. In response, I reduced the furosemide dose back to 80 mg daily.

Following this episode, I made no attempt at up-titration for a further month to allow recovery from the chest infection. Unfortunately Mrs A's symptoms did not return to her pre-holiday level and therefore she was now assessed at NYHA Class III. Mrs A now experienced fatigue throughout the day and was dyspnoeic with activities around her home although the dyspnoea did abate quickly with rest.

I decided to attempt the up-titration of her bisoprolol in the hope of gaining some symptomatic benefit at a higher dose. This proved to be a slow process and it took six months to reach the target dose of 10 mg daily. The first three dose increments proved to be problematic. Four days after the increase to 2·5 mg, Mrs A reported an increase in her level of dyspnoea. She had no obvious peripheral oedema and her weight was unchanged. She did however feel that her ankles were "tight and stiff". Her blood pressure was 90/50 mmHg. I took no action at this point. Unfortunately three days later her symptoms worsened and her weight increased by 1·5 kg. I now increased the dose of furosemide by 40 mg. With hindsight I should have increased the diuretic dose sooner. It took a further week for her weight to return to baseline and for Mrs A to feel an improvement in symptoms. The next two up-titrations evoked similar problems. I increased the dose of furosemide promptly before any obvious signs of fluid retention were present. The worsening symptoms were transient. After three days I was able to reduce the diuretic dose. Fortunately, the last two dose increments to 7·5 mg then 10 mg proved not to be problematic. Mrs A's pulse progressively slowed during the uptitration process from 80 to 66 bpm. Blood pressure, although persistently low, did not alter with the incremental increases.

Key issues arising from this case

Mrs A's renal function remained stable throughout all medication changes. The short-term increases in furosemide have not led to a significant rise in urea; it was previously elevated on a continuously higher dose of diuretic. I highlighted Mrs A's high cholesterol earlier. She was prescribed simvastatin for one month as her cholesterol rose to 8·5 mmol/l. Unfortunately her liver function deteriorated so simvastatin was discontinued. At present with strict dietary modification her cholesterol is 6·3 mmol/l. Mrs A has no other lifestyle risk factors that may precipitate an ischaemic event.

Eighteen months after her heart failure diagnosis, Mrs A underwent a total hip joint replacement under general anaesthesia. Her cardiovascular state was stable throughout the procedure. The only medication change was a reduction in the bisoprolol dose from 10 mg to 7·5 mg in the post-operative period. Again she was hypotensive. This was probably due in part to the use of opiates to control her surgical pain. Following discharge I was able to up-titrate this back to the target dose of 10 mg.

I have attempted a further up-titration of Mrs A's captopril, increasing the bedtime dose to 25 mg. She was initially stable with this but has recently been experiencing some postural symptoms. I have therefore reduced the dose back to 12·5 mg. Her heart failure is presently stable with NYHA Class III symptoms.

Current pharmacotherapy

- captopril 12·5 mg three times daily
- bisoprolol 10 mg daily
- furosemide 80 mg daily
- spironolactone 25 mg daily.

Postscript

The missing drug that may be of benefit to Mrs A is digoxin, which might improve her blood pressure with its positive inotropic action and therefore allow further increases to her ACE inhibitor. This is being deliberated at present.

Case study 2: A reflective account of the needs of a 70-year-old man dying from heart failure

IONA MCKAY

Introduction

As discussed in more detail in Chapter 10, effectively meeting the palliative care needs of those patients unfortunate enough to be dying from end stage heart failure represents an area of clinical practice where there are many questions still to be answered. The nature of heart failure is such that the patient may have numerous acute exacerbations of their symptoms and feel well following treatment. With good education, and with optimisation and control of medications, it may be possible to maintain this well being for some time. The Glasgow Heart Failure Liaison Service strives to meet these needs for its patients by basing itself on evidenced-based research.[1]

So, how can we determine when the terminal stage of illness has been reached? Hanratty and colleagues identified the difficulty in determining the illness trajectory in heart failure.[2] In response, Ellershaw and Ward suggest that a patient with a poor prognosis will have the following characteristics:

- previous admissions with worsening heart failure
- no identifiable reversible precipitant
- receiving optimum tolerated conventional drugs
- deteriorating renal function (Ward also notes that a low serum sodium is a known indicator of poor prognosis[3])
- failure to respond within 2–3 days to appropriate changes in diuretic or vasodilator drugs.[4]

It is within this context that I will discuss the case of a 70-year-old man with end stage heart failure, whom I regularly visited at home for more than nine months. In doing so, I believe several questions arise that are relevant to the following case scenario.

- When is the decision made that treatment is failing and end stage failure is being reached?
- Who explains what this means to the patient and their family, and who should be involved in end of life care?
- Where should the patient be looked after? Options may range from acute hospital setting to hospice care to their own home.
- What resources will be required to ensure palliative care needs are met?

Clinical background

Mr B, a 70-year-old man, was admitted to the Glasgow service following acute admission to hospital with worsening heart failure. He has a long cardiac history and has been known to his cardiologist for many years. The key features of his medical history are as follows:

- acute myocardial infarction in 1982 – prior to this he was being treated for hypertension

- coronary artery bypass grafting to three vessels in 1983
- history of hypercholesterolaemia and moderately high body mass index.

Mr B's recent history included slow atrial fibrillation and chronic renal failure. An echocardiogram in April 2002 showed mild–moderate left ventricular systolic dysfunction. It also showed a moderately–severely impaired mitral valve that undoubtedly masks the severity of left ventricular systolic dysfunction. A repeat echocardiogram was carried out in July 2002 and this was described in a letter from the cardiologist to the general practitioner as showing moderate–severe left ventricular systolic dysfunction. The letter highlighted some of the numerous problems that made day to day management of this patient difficult (see below).

Management issues

In January 2003, the treating cardiologist explained to Mr B and his wife that his condition was becoming more difficult to treat with every hospital admission. This was mainly due to his poor response to the medications. Using Ellershaw and Ward's criteria, it was clear that Mr B's prognosis was poor. However, what makes Mr B's case different is that this "end stage" has persisted for more than seven months. I think it would be fair to say that everyone involved in Mr B's care has been surprised that he has survived for so long.

As noted, it was the cardiologist who first raised the issue of end stage heart failure and what implications this had for Mr B's future management and prognosis. I reinforced this message to the patient in his own home during a prolonged discussion with Mr B, his wife, and his daughter (his main carers) and initiated the following practical measures:

- home oxygen therapy through liaison with Mr B's general practitioner
- suggestion that Mr B sleep in a comfortable chair with his head on a table with a pillow in front in an effort to alleviate the symptoms of paroxysmal nocturnal dyspnoea
- involvement of the district nursing services to dress his legs which by this time were leaking fluid due to the presence of gross peripheral oedema
- assessment for lifting and handling aids to help his main carers (this was done through liaison with social services)
- link with a hospice for advice on analgesics and anti-anxiolitics.

I was also able to facilitate other interventions designed to assist both Mr B and his main carers. This involved consultation with social services to optimise their financial benefits, to supply home help and overnight support, and to assess what aids are available to help make things easier for the immediate carers.

A key question, of course, is where should this type of "palliation" take place? In this instance, Mr B and his carers were happy for him to be supported at home. Since January Mr B has had two admissions to hospital. The first was at the end of February. On this occasion he had a poor response to intravenous diuretic therapy, and his mood became very low when hospitalised for three weeks during this episode. When Mr B returned home, I spoke to him and his wife about putting an action plan in place at night when his anxiety was at its worst. With consent from his general practitioner, I suggested that Mr B took sublingual lorazepam to help him to relax and then put some practical measures in place that included:

- sitting upright
- putting on his oxygen therapy
- opening windows to allow more air to circulate
- taking additional morphine if needed.

Since this time, Mr B has only had one further admission to hospital lasting two days and requirung minimal treatment.

Current status

Since his admission to hospital in March 2003, Mr B's medications have been changed. His diuretic therapy has been changed to torasemide 60 mg twice daily, which is a large volume of loop diuretic. Unfortunately this dosage now has little effect. Mr B has a package of care from social services, which includes home help services and overnight care. The district nurses visit three times a week to dress his legs, but the bandaging unfortunately makes mobility even more difficult. The nurse specialist from his local hospice visits occasionally, mainly to check that he is happy to have his care continued at home.

Through a lot of persuasion, Mr B has now had a urinary catheter inserted. This was essentially a measure designed to assist his wife and daughter with his care. They are both concerned that he may fall over when they stand him up from the chair to use a urinal. The patient initially saw this as another activity of daily living that was being taken away from him. He did however acknowledge and appreciate the concerns of his wife and his daughter. Mr B no longer requires oxygen therapy regularly and only uses it when he feels anxious. His main problems now are gross peripheral oedema and anxiety at night causing sleep deprivation. He sleeps a maximum of one to two hours at any one time. Surprisingly, however, Mr B still has a good appetite. End stage heart failure often precipitates cardiac cachexia that results in muscle mass loss. This muscle wasting can make symptoms of fatigue and breathlessness seem worse. Maintaining adequate nutrition is essential and, despite a slow weight loss, the fact that Mr B's good appetite has persisted is encouraging.

Future plans

We are considering using a subcutaneous infusion of furosemide in an attempt to help relieve his bilateral pitting oedema. This is a relatively new idea, which has been used with successful results. I discussed this with Mr B's cardiologist who is happy for us to go ahead with this treatment. To effectively manage Mr B at home highlights the importance of the multidisciplinary team being involved. I therefore discussed Mr B's management at the palliative care multidisciplinary meeting held weekly at the hospital. The palliative care consultant also suggested using caltostat dressings to his legs. This is a dressing used to treat patients with lymphoedema. It helps to return the fluid from the tissues back into the circulatory system. This will of course need to be done cautiously to prevent worsening symptoms of heart failure and he therefore suggested dressing one leg at time, initially using light compression. He also suggested using levomepromazine to help his anxiety and insomnia.

A meeting was then arranged with the general practitioner, district nurse, social worker, and myself to discuss the changes in Mr B's management and how best to implement them. During this meeting the district nurse highlighted that the patient had been in a lot of pain when the dressings to his legs were changed, and therefore his pain relief requires to be reassessed. A decision was also made regarding invasive procedures, for example checking blood chemistry, which was inappropriate at this stage of Mr B's illness.

The following changes were made to Mr B's treatment:

- commence subcutaneous furosemide infusion
- stop oral torasemide 120 mg daily
- commence cyclizine 50 mg three times daily
- stop oral oramorph
- commence MST 30 mg 12 hourly
- commence sevredol for breakthrough pain
- commence levomepromazine 6·25 mg in the evening.

To initiate these changes requires support from the general practitioner as well as the district nurses to change the furosemide syringe daily and to dress his legs with the caltostat dressing.

Key issues arising from this case study

Interdisciplinary teamwork and interagency collaboration are now widely recognised as a necessity in providing effective health and social care. Finlay and colleagues suggest there are three models of teamwork. These are: the hierarchical team, the parallel team, and the collaborative team.[5]

Finlay describes the parallel team as autonomous professionals dealing within their own specialist area, loosely linking with other members of the team when necessary (for example with the general practitioner, district nurses, and sometimes other services). The collaborative team knows each other well and works together closely on projects.

I would suggest that the care of Mr B has resulted in the combination of parallel and collaborative teamwork. On a day to day basis we work alongside one another with most communication being by telephone. On reflection, it is apparent to me that the central figures in the patient care are Mr B and his wife, who are providing the best communication to all parties involved. Initially I felt I was failing them; particularly by not knowing everything that was happening all the time. However, on critical reflection and discussion with Mr B and his wife, I can now see they have empowered themselves. Mr B's wife, in particular, has empowered herself to have much more confidence in her own abilities in caring for her husband.

This situation requires not only interdisciplinary teamwork, but also interagency collaboration, which potentially can make communication even harder. The main agencies involved in this case are:

- the primary care team (i.e. the general practitioner and district nursing services)
- social services – Mr B's care has been coordinated through one social worker which has been helpful
- a local hospice which is a charitable organisation
- a specialist heart failure nurse (myself) who is part of the primary care team working from secondary care to allow for effective liaison with cardiology specialists.

It is interesting to note that one person commented to me that we couldn't expect to do much more for this man because he already has "a fabulous package of care". This may be so, but in my opinion there can always be improvements that do not necessarily require additional expenditure: for example, the recent change in Mr B's medication to levomepromazine during the night which alleviated his nausea and insomnia. This action enabled the general practitioner to discontinue his temazepam, cyclizine, and domperidone – an important development in the face of significant polypharmacy.

Hanratty and colleagues suggest that doctors are keen to develop the role of the nurse in terminal heart failure. They say

> an often superior ability of the nurse is to liaise with other specialties and to communicate with the patients ... A nurse with expertise in cardiac palliative care is ideally placed to act as a co-ordinator of services, as well as influencing medical practice.[2]

At the moment I see myself as a nurse with expertise in heart failure management going through a rapid learning curve in palliative care management for this patient group. I have had feedback from palliative care specialists highlighting the differences in looking after this patient group due to the already mentioned difficulty in determining the trajectory of the illness. As discussed in Chapter 10, with the increasing prevalence of heart failure, I believe this is a role the heart failure nurse specialist is well placed to assume. It is natural for heart failure nurses to want to be involved in the terminal care of patients such as Mr B.

I would suggest that the fact that Mr B has survived longer than expected has allowed me to explore different options for care and improve communications with all of the agencies involved. Improving quality of services in health and social care is at the forefront of the health and social care agenda of the UK government. I would suggest that the real question is who determines "best quality" or "best value". In this new area of palliative care in heart failure, information on current practice needs to be collected to determine whether something is "best" practice or not and what possible changes can be made. I would suggest that a central figure in gathering this information has to be the patient's main carer (see Appendix 3), in this case the patient's wife. She has had contact with all the agencies involved and knows what has worked and what hasn't.

I believe that resources have been good in this particular case, mainly due to the excellent input from social services in organising home support. The overnight care helped to prevent Mr B's wife from becoming exhausted through lack of sleep, and subsequently more able to cope through the day. I feel that my role has changed somewhat, and that my visits mainly offer psychological support, probably more for his wife than for Mr B himself. Unfortunately due to other patient commitments I am usually only able to visit once a week. However I feel this has been sufficient for the carers and me to build up a good relationship and for them to put their trust in me to sort out day to day practical problems by communicating on their behalf with the other agencies involved.

Hopefully, the four major discussion points initially presented in this case study have been addressed in some way.

When is the decision made that treatment is failing and that end stage failure is being reached?

In this case it would appear that the criteria proposed by Ellershaw and Ward were of some use.[4]

Who explains what this means to the patient and their family, and who should be involved in end of life care?

It is very possible that failure of treatment will be noticed in the secondary care setting, and therefore one can assume that the most likely person to first address this issue with the patient will be the cardiologist. If however the patient is at home, this will necessitate general practitioner involvement. Clear guidance (for example as proposed by Ellershaw and Ward[4]) should be implemented to ensure continuity of care. Ideally guidelines would be implemented at national level to ensure best practice across the board. The heart failure nurse should play a pivotal role throughout in order to support the patient and their family through this difficult time. Reinforcement of information is essential. As such, there are three main components to good communication:

- active listening
- breaking bad news
- therapeutic dialogue[3]

Most nurses have had some form of training in developing good communication and informal counselling skills. I would suggest however that these naturally improve with nursing experience. I would also suggest that one of the main prerequisites to facilitate good communication is having time to listen.

From my experience with Mr B I believe everyone involved was essential to providing optimum care. I would, however, suggest that the role of the palliative care domiciliary nurse in many ways overlapped with the work I was doing. If specialist heart failure nurses were able to build their confidence and experience in this clinical setting, such duplication would not be necessary.

Where should palliation be applied?

The aforementioned is appropriate if the patient has opted for home care. Again, I believe that home care has been the best option in this case. If Mr B were in acute hospital care, it might be difficult to address all his palliative care needs and if he was in hospice care, particular attention to his heart failure management may be overlooked.

Finally, what resources will be required to ensure palliative needs are met?

I was surprised by the input required to optimise Mr B's care. I am sure the resources available are undoubtedly going to vary according to healthcare system. This has been a positive experience for me. All parties involved worked well together through good communication. Mr B's palliative care needs have been quite extensive and changed on a number of occasions over the last few months.

Postscript

In providing the care outlined above we undoubtedly improved Mr B's end of life experience by adhering to the basic principles of palliative care – good communication and close attention to symptom control in order to improve quality of remaining life. I hope that we can continue with this level of care and communication and make appropriate adjustments to Mr B's management in order to reach this goal and of course for his loved ones who will have their own period of reflection after his death.

References

1   Blue L, Lang E, McMurray JJ, *et al*. Randomised Controlled Trial of Specialist Nurse Intervention in Heart Failure. *BMJ* 2001;**323**:715–8.
2   Hanratty B, Hibbert D, Mair F, *et al*. Doctors' perceptions of palliative care for heart failure: focus study group. *BMJ* 2002;**325**:929–32.
3   Ward C, The Need for Palliative Care in the Management of Heart Failure. *Heart* 2002;**87**:294–8.
4   Ellershaw J, Ward C. Care of the dying patient: the last hours or days of life. *BMJ* 2003;**326**:30–4.
5   Finlay L. The challenge of working in teams. In: Brechin A, Brown H, Eby MA, eds. *Critical Practice in Health and Social Care*. London: Sage, 2000.

Case study 3: Management of a 45-year-old man with alcoholic cardiomyopathy

LAURA MACKINTOSH

Clinical background

This case study relates to Mr C, a 45-year-old man with an 18-year history of excess alcohol intake. As a result, he developed alcohol related cardiomyopathy and alcoholic liver disease (ALD). Mr C has also had frequent left sided pleural effusions which, following extensive investigation including thoracoscopy and biopsy, revealed the presence of inflammatory exudates only. He has chronic lymphoedema of his legs with keratinous skin changes and occasional ulcers. He is clinically obese with a body mass index of 38 kg/m². There is, however, no history of ischaemic heart disease, hyperlipidaemia, or hypertension. Echocardiography demonstrated that Mr C's left atrium, mitral valve and aortic valve are normal. His left ventricle is dilated and there is a large segment which is dyskinetic.

Current clinical and social status

Currently, Mr C has bilateral leg oedema that extends to his groin. He has moderate ascites and pitting oedema to a small sacral pad. His JVP is raised and he has a resting tachycardia of 100 bpm. Blood pressure is 120/60 mmHg. Mr C is breathless after walking 25 metres on the flat. He finds bathing and dressing difficult and is currently assessed as NYHA Class III. Fortunately, Mr C does not report paroxysmal nocturnal dyspnoea or orthopnoea.

Mr C lives with his wife and three children. They live in an inner city area where overall social deprivation, crime, unemployment, and intravenous drug use are high. The quality of housing is poor and local facilities are limited. Mr C has been unemployed for a number of years due to the decline in his health through ALD and his related cardiomyopathy. His wife is a carer for another family member who is terminally ill. Mr C is currently drinking but does attend Alcoholics Anonymous meetings and has an individual alcohol counsellor. He has had long periods of abstinence from alcohol and is keen to "give up for good". Mr C states that what makes it very hard for him to stop drinking is that his drinking partners are all good friends.

Mr C has lived with his diagnosis for some years now and is used to altering his medications to suit his symptoms. At times he is reluctant to carry out instructions or take guidance from healthcare professionals.

Current treatment/management plan

- lansoprazole 30 mg daily
- ferrous Sulphate 200 mg three times daily
- vitamin B Compound Strong 2 tablets three times daily
- thiamine 100 mg daily
- spironolactone 75 mg daily
- furosemide 120 mg twice daily
- slow K 600 mg twice daily.

The current treatment plan is to try to reintroduce an ACE inhibitor. Previous attempts failed due to dizziness. Once a reasonable dose of ACE inhibitor is achieved the plan is to then introduce a β-blocker; this would be a new therapeutic strategy in Mr C's case.

Prioritised clinical and social issues in Mr C's case

There are a number of important clinical and social issues that need to be addressed in this case that include:

- poor adherence
- excess fluid retention
- introduction and titration of an ACE inhibitor and β-blocker
- continued alcohol excess
- actions to address these issues.

Adherence

Education about his condition enabled Mr C to identify his symptoms and to intiate a self-management plan to help alleviate them. Information was provided about the reasons why we would wish to know about changes in his condition and why it was necessary to monitor his renal function. Time was given for Mr C to ask questions and digest the information. Subsequently it was negotiated with Mr C that he agreed to contact the heart failure nurses or his general practitioner if he thought his symptoms changed or deteriorated or if he had altered his medication regime.

Fluid excess

Initially Mr C's spironolactone was increased to 100 mg once daily (because of his liver disease and associated congestion) and his Slow K was stopped. This had a limited effect on fluid retention, so metolazone 2·5 mg on alternate days was added for two weeks, with twice weekly monitoring of renal function. This dosage certainly improved fluid retention and, although ascites and sacral oedema resolved, the bilateral oedema to the groin persisted. Mr C's renal function was stable. At this point it was suggested that Mr C go to hospital for intravenous therapy, but he refused to be admitted to hospital because he felt improved and could walk around 120 metres rather than 25. Instead, his spironolactone was increased to 200 mg per day and his furosemide was increased to 160 mg twice daily. Mr C's other treatment was left unchanged. Again renal function was monitored twice weekly and, surprisingly, remained stable.

Unfortunately, Mr C's fluid retention deteriorated again, ascites and sacral oedema returned, and a pleural effusion developed. Mr C was adamant that he was only drinking around 1 litre of fluid per day and that he had also stopped drinking alcohol. Mr C continued to refuse to be admitted to hospital. He then developed paroxysmal nocturnal dyspnoea. In response, his metolazone was increased to 5 mg per day and renal function was monitored twice weekly. Again renal function, surprisingly, remained stable.

Despite the huge amounts of oral diuretic there was no impact on fluid retention, probably due to poor absorption through his intestine. Mr C agreed to be admitted to hospital for intravenous therapy (at this point he was bordering NYHA Class IV). Mr C was in hospital for two weeks and a dry weight was achieved. He was discharged at this point and an ACE inhibitor and β-blocker were to be introduced in the community. Mr C was taking 80 mg of furosemide twice daily and spironolactone 200 mg once daily. His other medications remained the same (apart from Slow K which had been stopped prior to this admission).

ACE inhibitor and β-blocker titration

At this point ramipril 1·25 mg once daily was added to Mr C's regimen. His blood pressure and renal function were stable. After two weeks, his ramipril was increased to 1·25 mg twice daily and his blood pressure and renal function remained stable. After a further two weeks, his ramipril was increased to 2·5 mg twice daily. In response, Mr C's blood pressure dropped slightly to 110/60 from 120/60 mmHg. There were no reported symptoms of dizziness. Mr C then developed some ankle oedema and increased breathlessness. Furosemide was increased to 120 mg twice daily and his ramipril titration was temporarily put on hold. After two weeks the oedema had resolved and breathing pattern had returned to normal. At this point medical staff decided to try to introduce a β-blocker rather than increase his ramipril further whilst his diuretics were left at the increased dose. We waited a further two weeks before introducing the β-blocker. Thus Mr C had one month without medication change. Then bisoprolol at 1·25 mg once daily was added to his treatment. After two weeks this was increased to 2·5 mg once daily. Fluid retention and renal function were stable but his blood pressure dropped to 100/60 mmHg.

Alcohol excess

Despite having many months of abstinence Mr C resumed drinking alcohol at this point. No further titrations have been made to medication or treatment. We have been unable to contact him and when we do make contact he is either drunk or fails to answer the door. His wife has encouraged him to re-establish contact with his alcohol counsellor without success.

Postscript

At this point we are unable to monitor Mr C's condition and adjust his treatment accordingly. If it were possible, we would attempt to further up-titrate his β-blocker and ACE inhibitor. We would also encourage him to return to Alcoholics Anonymous and re-establish contact with his alcohol counsellor.

Case study 4: Managing heart failure of unknown aetiology in a 48-year-old woman

LINDA MCGINNIS

Clinical background

This case study relates to Mrs D, a 48-year-old woman who was admitted to hospital with increasing breathlessness and orthopnoea over three days prior to admission. She had ankle swelling for two weeks prior to this and her general practitioner commenced her on furosemide 20 mg once daily. On admission her ECG showed left bundle branch block. On clinical examination she had bi-basal crepitations, raised JVP to her ears, and peripheral oedema to ankle level. She was treated with intravenous diuretics and her condition improved.

Before the removal of a benign brain tumor (cerebro pontine angle meningioma), Mrs D did have an ECG performed last year that showed no abnormalities. Prior to this, she had no other significant past medical history other than alcohol abuse. A troponin level was checked to exclude an ischaemic event and this was normal. There was however derangement of her liver function tests. She had an echocardiogram performed, which showed a globally impaired dilated left ventricle with moderate to severe left ventricular impairment, a dilated left atrium, mild mitral regurgitation, and mild tricuspid regurgitation.

A diagnosis of cardiomyopathy was made. The cause of her underlying cardiomyopathy was possibly alcohol abuse. Mrs D's alcohol abuse was nearly 10 years ago when she was drinking at least two bottles of vodka over a day. She stated this was only over a period of six months following the accidental death of her child at the age of 18 years. Her differential diagnosis would be idiopathic cardiomyopathy. However, Mrs D continues to demonstrate abnormal liver function tests and her GGT is over 200 micromol/l.

First home visit

I visited Mrs D within a week of her discharge from hospital. She felt well and was stable. Her medical therapy included captopril 25 mg three times per day and furosemide 40 mg once daily.

Her chest was clear and she had no ankle oedema or visible JVP. Apart from educational intervention she did not require any active intervention at this point in time.

Subsequent management

In the following week (two weeks post discharge) Mrs D developed ankle swelling, increasing breathlessness, a weight gain of 2 kg, and orthopnoea. As a result of this clinical deterioration, she was readmitted to hospital. Unfortunately she was taken to another local hospital. During this episode she was an inpatient for three days and required intravenous diuretics. Following this hospital admission her ACE inhibitor was changed to an equivalent dose of ramipril and her furosemide was increased from 40 mg to 80 mg daily.

I continued to follow Mrs D's management within a few days from her discharge from hospital. On this visit Mrs D said she did not feel well and said she was feeling very dizzy at times. She was hypotensive (96/60 mmHg) but this was her normal blood pressure since discharge and she also had a tachycardia of 120 bpm (sinus rhythm) – her previous heart rate being around 90 bpm. She also complained of increasing breathlessness (equivalent to NYHA Class II). As a result, I decided to split the dose of her ACE inhibitor (ramipril) from 7·5 mg once daily to 5 mg in the morning and 2·5 mg in the evening. I also arranged for her to have an early clinic review with a cardiologist.

By the time of her clinic review Mrs D's dizziness had improved. The cardiologist increased her ramipril to 5 mg twice daily. Her chest was clear and she was free of ankle swelling. However, her JVP still remained elevated and it was decided she was not stable enough to be considered for a β-blocker at this time.

Mrs D remained stable for another two weeks then once again developed ankle swelling, had a weight gain of a 1–2 kg, and became markedly orthopnoeic requiring three to four pillows to sleep at night. On clinical examination, she had bi-basal crepitations and slight ankle swelling, and her JVP was raised nearly to her ears. In this instance I was inclined to increase her furosemide. However, her potassium was 3·2 mmol/l and I routinely sought medical advice as part of our guidelines in the instance of abnormal electrolyte results. I therefore contacted Mrs D's cardiologist who advised me to double her furosemide from 80 mg once daily to twice daily and also request her general practitioner to prescribe potassium supplements. I then re-evaluated her blood chemistry in one week. Her potassium had increased to 4·8 mmol/l during this period. Following discussion with her cardiologist, it was decided to stop her potassium supplements but leave her on an increased dose of diuretic as she was feeling less breathless.

Mrs D's symptoms have now stabilised but her potassium levels continue to be labile. On discontinuation of her potassium supplements her potassium levels fell and she once again required supplementation.

Current status

Over the past three weeks Mrs D's weight has been steady, her chest is clear, she has no ankle oedema. Her JVP continues to be elevated but improved at a height of 6 cm. She is on maximum dose of ramipril but, unfortunately, she is not yet stable enough to commence a β-blocker. If she remains stable, I plan to decrease her furosemide back to her original dose of 80 mg once daily. If her potassium levels stabilise, the potassium supplements will be discontinued. Her liver function tests remain abnormal. Both the consultant and I are unsure if she has stopped taking alcohol, and her consultant is unsure as to why this may be.

Postscript

The cause of Mrs D's cardiomyopathy is still unknown and clearly hindering definitive management. Further investigation of her liver abnormalities is planned, as is a coronary angiogram to exclude the possibility of underlying ischaemic heart disease.

Case study 5: The difficulty in managing end stage heart failure in a 68-year-old man

KIRSTIE MOWAT

Clinical background

This case study relates to Mr E, a 68-year-old man who was initially managed by my colleague for four months until she left the service and I took over his care. During this period he had four previous admissions to hospital with decompensated heart failure. All of these admissions occurred outside the working hours of the Heart Failure Liaison Service which operates Monday to Friday 9.30 am to 5.30 pm. His past clinical history is extensive and includes: ischaemic heart disease for over twenty years; a coronary artery bypass graft (1983), an aortic valve replacement (1989), complete heart block and required a permanent pacemaker (1994). A thallium scan (1997) showed a large dilated heart with poor overall myocardial perfusion and estimated ejection fraction of 29%. During his last hospital admission he had an echocardiogram that confirmed severe left ventricular systolic dysfunction.

In spite of this extensive history, Mr E continued to smoke and drink alcohol on a social basis. Mr E was a retired machine operator and lived with his wife who was very supportive. They have two children living away from home. Mr E's first admission with decompensated heart failure was in 2001. When I initially met Mr E and his wife, they did not feel they required input from outside agencies. However, they were unsure if they were receiving adequate financial benefits and I referred Mr E and his wife to social services for assessment.

First home visit

Mr E was a very frail gentleman who had a reasonable understanding of his condition and the symptoms he was experiencing. His wife was present, and took the lead when I asked any questions. She also took the lead to inform me of his progress and his current health status, although I directed my questions to Mr E. He gave the impression of being tired of life in general.

He was NYHA Class IV, dyspnoeic at rest, bilateral leg oedema to knee level, mild ascites. His appetite was poor, although his fluid intake was adequate. His sleeping pattern was poor and he described symptoms of paroxysmal nocturnal dyspnoea overnight and was waking several times to micturate. He was jaundiced in appearance. Blood pressure was stable at 100/70 mmHg, pulse 70 bpm, weight 64 kg.

Drug therapy

- furosemide 120 mg twice daily
- enalapril 20 mg twice dail
- warfarin 2 mg once daily
- simvastatin 20 mg evening
- allopurinol 100 mg once daily
- lactulose 10 ml twice daily
- bendrofluazide 10 mg once daily, which had been started three days prior to my visit, during his last hospital admission.

The β-blocker he had previously been taking was bisoprolol. This had been changed to carvedilol during his last hospital admission, and subsequently stopped by his cardiologist as he felt this was aggravating his heart failure symptoms. He had previously been taking spironolactone but this also had to be discontinued due to Mr E developing significant renal dysfunction.

Management plan

Mr E was still significantly fluid overloaded despite taking a large dose of loop diuretic and a thiazide diuretic. I therefore sought advice from the contact cardiologist. Prior to this I checked his blood chemistry – renal function was similar to previous results: sodium 138 mmol/l, potassium 3·7 mmol/l, urea 15·7 mmol/l, and creatinine 170 micromol/l. Due to his jaundiced appearance I also checked liver function tests, which were normal apart from an elevation in alkaline phosphatase thought to be due to hepatic congestion. Following discussion with the cardiologist he advised that Mr E continue with bendrofluazide 10 mg once daily for another three days and then to review the situation.

When I visited Mr and Mrs E three days later he had improved significantly. He remained NYHA Class IV but was less fatigued, dyspnoea had improved, oedema had reduced to ankle level, and ascites had resolved. His sleeping pattern had not improved, but he did not complain of orthopnoea. There was a further weight loss of 2·5 kg, blood pressure was 90/50 mmHg and pulse 76 bpm. I rechecked blood chemistry to monitor the effect of the thiazide diuretic (see Chapter 9 section on thiazide diuretics); renal function remained unchanged. It now seemed appropriate to reduce the thiazide diuretic, and therefore I consulted the cardiologist and this was agreed and the dose of bendrofluazide was reduced to 5 mg once daily.

I visited Mr E one week later and his condition remained stable. He had a further weight loss of 1·5 kg (now 60 kg) and reduction in ankle oedema; vital signs and renal function were similar to the previous week. He did however remain tired and dyspnoeic at rest and I was concerned that he was orthopnoeic and experiencing symptoms of paroxysmal nocturnal dyspnoea. I asked him if he was waking up breathless or did he have a cough? He continued to say this was not the case, but his wife expressed concern about how breathless he was overnight. Mr E appeared very anxious.

I spoke to his general practitioner and asked whether he would consider prescribing sedation to help the patient to relax. He was reluctant to prescribe a mild opiate without seeing the patient and arranged to visit Mr E the following day. I planned to visit Mr E the following week. Unfortunately, prior to my visit he was readmitted to hospital with deteriorating heart failure. This admission was once again outside the hours of the Heart Failure Liaison Service.

End stage management

During this admission he required inotropic support. His renal function deteriorated significantly following intravenous diuretics, and he became symptomatically hypotensive. The dose of furosemide was reduced to 80 mg twice daily and the dose of enalapril reduced to 10 mg twice daily. The cardiologist discussed his prognosis with both Mr E and his wife, explaining that there was further deterioration in his condition and he was not responding to medical therapy and therefore symptom control was now the main aim of care. Mr E decided to take early discharge from hospital as he wanted to spend as much time at home as possible. The hospital initiated a package of community care to facilitate this.

I visited Mr E at home two days later. Although he remained anxious and frightened, he was now able to discuss his fears with me. He requested a change in night sedation as he found the benzodiazepine (temazepam) that his general practitioner had prescribed to be ineffective. Mrs E asked if I would be able to get her husband a wheelchair to allow her to take him out if he felt able. I was able to access this through a local charitable organisation that provided equipment for short term use in patients with terminal illness. District nursing staff were coming in twice daily to attend to personal care and to provide additional support for Mrs E.

I felt it was now an appropriate time to ask Mr E what his wishes were should his symptoms deteriorate further. Did he want to go back into hospital or would he prefer to be at home? He was quite clear he wanted to stay at home and to die at home. His wife was very quiet during this conversation and she had obvious concerns. She subsequently told me that when he became breathless at night she panicked and called the emergency services or took him to the emergency room herself – hence the pattern of recurrent readmissions. This would explain the admissions to hospital that were occurring outside the hours of the Heart Failure Liaison Service. I tried to reassure her and, as an additional supportive measure, I suggested that a referral to the local hospice might be helpful. She said she would discuss this with Mr E.

Their general practitioner visited the following day and made a referral to the local hospice. I visited Mr E again a few days later and his condition had deteriorated further. He was symptomatically worse and increasingly breathless at rest. Home oxygen had been supplied and he was using this almost continuously. He was frightened to go to sleep and he was now expectorating white frothy sputum. He was also becoming increasingly confused and was having difficulty swallowing his medication. The district nurses were in attendance overnight to allow Mrs E some rest. I arranged a visit for Mr E from the out of hours general practitioner service, but prior to this an ambulance was called following an emergency call by his wife. He died shortly after this without reaching hospital.

Postscript

What have I learned from this experience and what can we do to prevent this happening again?

There are always going to be difficult situations that arise, particularly with a service that only operates on a Monday to Friday basis. I see no easy answers. Certainly it is clear that we need to develop relationships with palliative care services so that we can access advice for our patients at the end of their life and make decisions with them that are right for them. There need to be clearly documented pathways of care that can be used by all professionals visiting the home so that out-of-hours staff are aware of the desires and wishes of the patient and his family.

Case study 6: An account of a patient's journey following a diagnosis of left ventricular systolic dysfunction of ischaemic aetiology

YVONNE MILLERICK

Introduction

This case study maps the journey of a patient and his family following a diagnosis of chronic heart failure secondary to left ventricular systolic dysfunction. It outlines the personal, medical, nursing, and social needs, and highlights the wider implications of heart failure and its progression.

Background

Mr F is 58 years old and has worked all his life as a welder until he was forced to take early retirement two years ago due to ill health. To date he has had several admissions to hospital during which time he was diagnosed with hypertension, type II diabetes, ischaemic heart disease, hyperlipidaemia, and atrial fibrillation, and required to have a coronary artery bypass graft.

Mr F presented to hospital in July 2002 with increasing breathlessness and chest pain. This was the first time he presented with symptoms suggestive of heart failure. He had bilateral thigh oedema and a raised jugular venous pressure of approximately 8 cm. The liver was enlarged 4 finger breadths and was pulsatile. Other symptoms included fatigue, orthopnoea, paroxysmal nocturnal dyspnoea, and a dry hacking cough which had developed over the last 10 days. Prior to hospital admission his pharmacological regime included furosemide 80 mg once daily, digoxin 250 microg once daily, warfarin as directed by the anticoagulation clinic, simvastatin 20 mg nightly, and human mixtard 30/70 two injections daily. He had a number of investigations including an electrocardiogram, which confirmed atrial fibrillation but showed no new evidence of a recent myocardial infarction, a chest *x* ray film, which showed pulmonary congestion and an enlarged heart, and an echocardiogram, which confirmed moderately impaired left ventricular systolic dysfunction. Blood pressure was 105/60 mmHg and heart rate was irregular at approximately 80 beats per minute. Mr F remained in hospital for seven days during which time his condition stabilised following intravenous diuretics. Pre-discharge blood chemistry was stable, urea 9 mmol/l, creatinine 110 mmol/l, haemoglobin 12 g/dl (international ratio 2·2). Mr F was referred to the Heart Failure Liaison Service for post discharge follow up.

First home visit

I visited Mr F at home four days after hospital discharge. He lives at home with his wife in a first floor flat with fourteen stairs to its main door. His wife works part time five nights per week and looks after their one-year-old granddaughter from 9am to 3pm Monday to Friday as well as being the main carer for her husband. They also have three married daughters who are busy working mothers.

My first impression of Mr F was that he was an ill looking man who appeared much older than his 58 years. Following a brief introduction about my role and the service aims it was apparent that both Mr F and his wife were keen to have the support of the service and were willing to learn and actively participate in the care planning. I took time to explain the term heart failure and associated symptoms. I realised that both Mr F and his wife had very limited knowledge and understanding of heart failure and were only beginning to make sense of what had been happening prior to this hospital admission. I used this opportunity to relate Mr F's symptoms to his condition and to enhance his understanding further. Education is an integral part of care delivery; a lack of patient or family education has been linked to hospital readmission.

Mr F was breathless on minimal exertion and was finding it difficult to hold a conversation without stopping for breath. He also gave a history of experiencing paroxysmal nocturnal dyspnoea and was requiring an additional two pillows to enhance his sleeping pattern. On examination he had bilateral pitting calf oedema, which had deteriorated following hospital discharge; he also had evidence of mild abdominal ascites. When I asked him about these symptoms, he felt that there had been no change over the last few days. As a heart failure specialist nurse, it is important to remember that my assessment of symptoms has been enhanced by my professional knowledge. Mr F and his wife can only base their assessment on their own experience (what they see and how they feel).

The overt symptoms that were so obvious to me were less obvious to Mr F and his wife. It is for this reason that I relate my assessment to patients' daily activities. I noticed that he was not wearing socks or slippers and when I asked him if he felt that they were tight and uncomfortable he mentioned that he had been unable to wear them over the last couple of days. I also noticed that he had pyjama trousers on with a shirt and when I asked him about this he told me that his trousers had become too tight and he was unable to fasten them at the waist. This again had only occurred over the last couple of days. By highlighting the connection between subtle changes in symptoms and problems with daily activities I was hoping to improve both Mr F's and his wife's knowledge and therefore enhance their assessment skills and overall management.

Tiredness and muscle weakness in chronic heart failure are thought to be related to the changes that occur in skeletal muscle structure and function, impairing the muscle blood flow and endothelial function. Mr F was having difficulty with activities of daily living and was relying heavily on his wife to help him wash and dress each day. He was managing to walk the short distance from his bedroom to the living room each morning. However once he sat down he found it very difficult to get up from his chair. The inconvenience of his diuretic therapy required him to use a urinal to urinate, as he was unable to get to the toilet. Symptoms and exercise capacity are used to grade the severity of heart failure and to some extent are used as a predictor of treatment. The measurement tool used to determine classification of symptoms is the New York Heart Association scale commonly referred to as NYHA Class I–IV. As Mr F is unable to carry out any physical activity without symptoms and is breathless at rest he is classed as NYHA IV.

Initial management plan

Mr F was discharged home with a number of medication changes that had caused him some concern and confusion. He commented that the dose of furosemide had been doubled to 80 mg twice daily. However as this had never been explained to him he assumed it was an error and decided to revert to the original pre-admission dose of 80 mg once daily. I suspected at this stage that this innocent action by Mr F had resulted in the deterioration of his heart failure symptoms. I advised Mr F and his wife that careful monitoring of diuretic therapy was required to prevent over-treatment and that it was important to report symptoms of thirst, flaky skin, dizziness, feeling generally "washed out", or difficulty passing urine. I explained that achieving and maintaining a dry weight may require frequent diuretic dose changes, and also advised that the timing of the diuretic need not be fixed and could be changed in response to the daily routine. By explaining about a flexible diuretic regime I hoped to increase Mr F's awareness of the importance of diuretic compliance.

During his hospital admission Mr F was commenced on a small dose of ramipril 2·5 mg once daily. Carvedilol was also introduced at 3·125 mg twice daily. His other medication, which included digoxin, simvastatin, warfarin, and human mixtard 30/70, remained unchanged.

Further assessment and education with Mr F and his wife included discussion about daily weight and the importance of measuring this accurately on a daily basis. I advised Mr F and his wife that a weight gain or loss of 1–1·5 kg over a 48-hour period was significant and would need to be reported and acted on promptly. I provided a set of weighing scales. His weight had increased since his discharge from hospital by 2·5 kg and although variation can occur from one set of scales to another I felt that the overt symptoms of dyspnoea and peripheral oedema supported this change.

Although compliance with sodium and fluid restriction are very difficult to measure I advised Mr F and his wife about this. Mr F said that he liked to taste salt in his food and was understandably reluctant to change this. However I managed to persuade him to reduce his fluid intake from 3 litres to 2 litres daily initially and reduce the sodium intake by using herbs, spices, and lemon juice instead. I also advised him that there was evidence to suggest that restricting sodium and fluid daily could help to reduce peripheral oedema and therefore lead to a diuretic reduction. The thought of requiring less diuretic was very appealing to him.

Mr F was a non-smoker, limited his alcohol intake to four units twice weekly, received an annual flu immunisation and adhered well to his medication. He therefore had no other risk factors that required discussion at this stage. He gave consent for a social work assessment to ensure that he was receiving the maximum support available.

Subsequent management

In response to deteriorating symptoms and stable blood chemistry I advised Mr F to increase the dose of furosemide by 40 mg daily and increase the dose of ramipril. Both these changes were within the medical therapy guidelines used in our service and were agreed by his general practitioner. I arranged to visit Mr F at home in one week's time.

When I next visited Mr F he was feeling better. He was no longer breathless at rest, abdominal ascites had reduced, bilateral calf oedema had resolved to ankle level, and his weight had reduced by 1·5 kg. His blood chemistry and blood pressure were stable and I advised him to continue with the increased diuretic dose for a further three days and also to increase the dose of ramipril by a further 2·5 mg daily.

Mr F tolerated the increased dose of ramipril without adverse effect and his dose of diuretic was maintained at 80 mg once daily with no deterioration in symptoms. I decided to leave his medication unchanged and review him again in one month to increase the dose of carvedilol.

Two weeks later I received a telephone call from Mr F requesting a home visit. When I arrived he was looking very ill although his heart failure status was relatively stable. His main problems were symptoms of nausea, anorexia, extreme fatigue, and dizziness. He was bradycardic with a rate of 54 beats per minute and hypotensive at 88/60 mmHg. Nausea and anorexia had stopped him from taking his morning medication. I therefore checked a digoxin level and blood chemistry as I suspected that his symptoms were digoxin related. I explained to Mr F that he may not be tolerating the dose of digoxin and advised him that admission to hospital might be required depending on the blood results. I arranged to telephone him later that day when I knew his wife would be there to support him. The biochemist telephoned later that morning to confirm the digoxin level was 6 nmol/l and, following discussion with the cardiologist and general practitioner, hospital admission was arranged. Mr F was hospitalised for 10 days and the digoxin toxicity resolved but his symptoms of heart failure deteriorated. As a result furosemide was stopped and he was commenced on bumetanide 5 mg daily; digoxin was also re-introduced at the lower dose of 62·5 microg daily.

Following discharge Mr F required weekly visits for deteriorating heart failure symptoms and he was commenced on bendrofluazide 2·5 mg daily increasing to 5 mg. Unfortunately these symptoms persisted despite combined diuretic therapy of loop and thiazide. His blood chemistry remained stable. Following discussion with the cardiologist and general practitioner it was decided that spironolactone 25 mg should be added to his daily medication. He was also commenced on oromorph 2·5 mg at night as his sleeping pattern was badly affected with paroxysmal nocturnal dyspnoea and this was depressing both him and his wife.

Following this change of therapy I noticed he was quite distant towards me when I visited and I decided to mention it to him, whereupon he broke down in tears and told me that he was frightened that he would die in the house in front of his grandchild. The oromorph had triggered this reaction as he associated morphine with dying. This breakthrough led to an in-depth discussion and resulted in the formulation of a future management plan that was agreed by his family, general practitioner, and cardiologist. I also reassured him that the use of oromorph was effectively reducing his dyspnoea at night and was therefore enhancing his sleep pattern. Over the next month his heart failure symptoms improved and the dose of diuretic was reduced gradually to bendrofluazide 2·5 mg on

Mondays and Thursdays only and bumetanide 2 mg twice daily. Serum digoxin was within the therapeutic range so he was maintained on the lower dose of 62·5 microg daily. His blood chemistry had deteriorated slightly during this period (urea 17 mmol/l, creatinine 150 mmol/l), but this was still within the parameters outlined in the medical therapy guidelines on the use of spironolactone and he continued with this therapy. Following discussion with the cardiologist it was agreed to try and increase the dose of carvedilol as Mr F's symptoms had been stable for one month and both his blood pressure and heart rate were stable. Over the next six weeks I was able to increase the dose of carvedilol to 18·75 mg twice daily without adverse effect.

I telephoned Mr F as planned to review his symptoms following the increase in the dose of carvedilol from 12·5 mg twice daily to 18·75 mg twice daily, four days earlier. During our conversation he reported increasing dyspnoea and slight ankle oedema associated with a weight gain of 1 kg. In response to these symptoms I advised him to increase the dose of bumetanide by 1 mg daily for the next three days and continue with his other medications. I arranged to visit him on the fourth day.

He unfortunately did not respond to the increased diuretic and his symptoms of dyspnoea and ankle oedema persisted. His daily weight had also increased by a further 0·5 kg. Although he was haemodynamically stable I advised him to revert to the lower dose of carvedilol 12.5 mg twice daily. When I telephoned a week later his heart failure symptoms had stabilised. I therefore advised him to revert to the original dose of bumetanide (2 mg twice daily).

Current status

Mr F has been relatively stable for the last two months and continues to receive the support of the Heart Failure Liaison Service. His heart failure status fluctuates between NYHA Class III and IV and he is on the following therapy:

- bumetanide 2 mg twice daily
- bendrofluazide 2·5 mg Mondays and Thursdays only
- ramipril 5 mg twice daily
- carvedilol 12·5 mg twice daily
- spironolactone 25 mg once daily
- digoxin 62·5 microg once daily
- oromorph 2·5 mg at night
- simvastatin 20 mg at night
- warfarin as directed
- human mixtard 30/70 twice daily injections.

Mr F's compliance with medication, daily weight and risk factor modification is commendable. He is managing to get out of his flat a little more with the help of his wife and they are both benefiting from a home help twice weekly. Following the occupational assessment he has been provided with a walk-in shower and raised toilet seat. A new bed with elevated headrest has made a considerable difference to his sleeping pattern and although they are still waiting on a customised wheelchair they have been provided with a temporary one from a local charity. This has improved both his quality of life and that of his wife, as they are now able to go out as a couple again and be part of society.

Future management

Future management plans for Mr F will continue to be targeted at effective symptom control and open communication. Frequent changes to therapy in response to symptoms require trust, co-operation, and commitment from the patient, family, cardiologist, general practitioner, and the heart failure liaison nurse. If symptoms permit I will consider increasing the dose of carvedilol and/or combining the ramipril with an angiotensin-II receptor antagonist in response to the recent evidence from the CHARM study.

Postscript

Undoubtedly there will come a time when therapeutic options have been exhausted and a more appropriate management plan will be required which focuses on end of life issues and symptom palliation. Having already discussed these briefly I now know that when that time comes Mr F wishes to be admitted to hospital and be resuscitated. As a heart failure liaison nurse my goal of treatment will be to address the physical, psychological, social, spiritual, and cultural needs of my patient and his family in a compassionate and professional way.

Appendix 3: Supporting the caregiver in heart failure

JOHN CARSON

Introduction

A carer is someone who looks after a friend, relative, or neighbour who may be disabled, frail, or ill. The number of carers within any given community is enormous. For example, in a population of 5 million people, there are over 600 000 carers (one in five adults) in Scotland. Half of all carers give up work to care for someone thereby losing career and pension opportunities. One third of carers never receive a regular break or respite from their caring duties and two thirds say their own health has suffered as a result of caring responsibilities. Data presented at the 2003 European Society of Cardiology meeting demonstrates that those who care for someone with heart failure often have worse quality of life.[1]

It is estimated that Scotland's carers alone save the UK National Health Service £3·4 billion each year.[2] Care provided by informal caregivers contributes to the maintenance of dependent older people in the primary care setting. Without this contribution there would be a much greater burden imposed upon both the secondary care and social services. Given the relative cost-effectiveness of maintaining patients with heart failure in the community, as opposed to in long-term residential care or in acute care institutions,[3] the role of carers in heart failure is especially important.

Issues surrounding caregiver support

In recent years initiatives have been developed to help us strive towards adopting a more collaborative approach to treating patients. The emphasis has been increasingly put on delivering care in the primary care setting with strategies such as outreach programmes and early discharge, and community specialties such as heart failure, diabetes, and pulmonary liaison. With this approach an increased burden has been placed on primary care health professionals and also on the families of these patients.[1] It is often assumed that the responsibility of care has been readily accepted by the patient's family. However, this assumption, no matter how well intentioned, is often misplaced. Previous studies have highlighted the problems the burden of care on family members can cause, including strains put on physical and mental health, finances, and carer family time.[1,4–8]

Due to the nature of heart failure, the patients we see as part of the Glasgow Heart Failure Liaison Service are often elderly with poor mobility and other debilitating comorbidities. Consequently we often involve the family members to varying degrees in the implementation of some aspects of the patient's care. Importantly, the natural assumption that the carers will cope is not one that should be made readily without a discussion with the patient's family/carers. There are several tools for measuring the quality of life of caregivers of patients with cancer, which with little adaptation can be used for carers of all chronic disease sufferers. The caregiver quality of life index cancer scale (CQOLC), the caregiver quality of life index (CQLI), the quality of life tool (QOLT), and the quality of life index cancer version are all examples of tools used effectively in qualitative research to study the burdens faced by carers of cancer patients. They are all able to assess the physical, social, financial, and psychological dimensions of carers' family life.[9] Of the four instruments, the QOLT is perhaps the most suitable for nursing research and audit due to its brevity.

We should recognise also that the above strains on the caregiver could have a detrimental affect on the patient, who may be sensitive to the overt signs of stress and strain on that person. This, in turn, could lead to increased feelings of anxiety and worry that they are simply a burden and nothing much else to that person. It has been suggested that this can lead to unsuccessful adjustment to chronic disease and any subsequent caregiver relationship.[10] To provide effective care however the caregiver must have access to adequate resources to ensure that they do not suffer under the pressure of the burden of care.[3] Accessing this type of support can often be difficult and may involve having to plough through a myriad of bureaucracy to get the resources that they are due. It has been suggested in the past that the ability to access these resources is directly related to the empowerment and self-esteem felt by the caregiver.[11] Access to these resources needs to be provided for carers who may be less inclined to be proactive when dealing with support agencies or who perhaps do not benefit from having past experience of knowing how to get through what can sometimes seem like miles of red tape.

Supporting caregivers

Carers can resent the fact that their goodwill is exploited as a substitute for adequate levels of care provision to the person they care for. While most would like to maintain a caring input they would prefer to be in a position to choose the level and nature of involvement. There is therefore a need for agencies not to rely on carers but to guarantee basic service provision and work in partnership with the carer.

An important element of the supportive role of the specialist nurse, which perhaps has arisen by default, is as a facilitator for, and conduit to, such support agencies. The nurse can play an essential part in obtaining such things as increased home help, occupational therapy and social work support, befriending schemes, respite care, overnight carers, and day care facility to name a few. Patients and their carers may need a broad area of support and for the nurse to be able to help them access this support requires an equally broad knowledge of the services and agencies available. This can often only be gained through experience and often by "trial and error".

The extent of carer support will naturally vary on a regional basis. In Glasgow as in many other regions, there is not yet support specific for carers of heart failure patients other than the Glasgow service itself. However, there are many agencies providing "generic carer resources".

A collaboration has been formed between council, social work, charity, and health agencies in Glasgow to design a strategy for helping carers. The joint carers strategy 2002–2005 has been designed to improve supportive information for carers, improve local services that help carers cope, introduce helpful legislature, ensure national standards for respite breaks for carers, and ensure on an ongoing basis carers receive appropriate help.[12]

Results from a 2001 initiative, the Carers Legislation Working Group, should be of help to carers. This initiative now gives carers the right to request an independent carer assessment irrespective of whether the cared for person is being assessed by the local authority. At the time of reporting it was recognised that this was being underutilised and that there is a need for increasing the profile of this support.

The Greater Glasgow Primary Care National Health Service Trust also offers carers a support line and a booklet that was compiled as a joint venture with Health and Social Services as a response to carers' comments about the lack of information that was previously available to them. The West of Scotland Carers Forum is a national support collective which provides carers with support lines, literature, support groups and web-based information.[2] It also forms part of the Coalition of Carers in Scotland, which is a group formed to raise the awareness of carers' plight with politicians. It has supported the publication of the "Strategy for Carers in Scotland" and had success in helping to introduce changes in legislation in the *Health and Community Care (Scotland) Bill*. It was also a fundamental partner in the joint carers' strategy.

Conclusion

The Glasgow Joint Carers' Strategy highlights the current need for improving uptake of appropriate services for carers and also the need for "achieving greater co-ordination between health and social work particularly in identifying 'hidden carers' ". Glasgow has spent £1·3 million annually on running nine carer centres and projects across the city. It is impossible to estimate what percentage of carers are utilising them but it is recognised that at present it is probably not high enough. It should be a fundamental part of any primary care nurse specialist's role to avail themselves of at least some of the services and networks offered to support carers.

In being critical of our own practice, within the Glasgow Heart Failure Liaison Service we should perhaps strive to form closer links with social services to "streamline" the caregivers' access to social services and to compile more lean information on how to get support. As such, there is arguably a need for nurses and other healthcare professionals to have more formal education on the support available from social services. We should not seek to adopt the role of the social worker, but the specialist heart failure nurse, by the very nature of their work, is often best placed to ensure optimum outcomes are gained for the families. With this issue in mind, it is imperative that any heart failure service performs regular qualitative review of the life experience of patient carers to ensure they are coping and that they are being provided with effective support. Clearly, there is more scope for research in this area and the Glasgow service is investigating ways to facilitate more peer-group support for carers of patients enrolled in the service.

References

1   Luttik M, Jaarsma T, Van Veldhuisen DJ. Quality of life of caregivers is worse compared to patients with congestive heart failure. *Eur Heart J* 2003;**24**:64.
2   West of Scotland Carer's Forum. www.wscf.info/aboutus.htm (accessed Oct 2003).
3   Stewart S, Jenkins A, Buchan S, Capewell S, McGuire A, McMurray JJ. The current cost of heart failure to the National Health Service in the UK. *Eur J Heart Fail* 2002;**4**:361–71.
4   Kesby SG. Nursing care and collaborative practice. *J Clin Nurs* 2002;**11**:357–66.
5   Brostrom A, Stromberg A, Dahlstrom U, Fridlund B. Congestive heart failure, spouses' support and the couple's sleep situation: A critical incident technique analysis. *J Clin Nurs* 2003;**12**:223–33.
6   Mastrian KG, Ritter C, Deimling GT. Predictors of caregiver health strain. *Home Health Nurse* 1996;**14**:209–17.
7   Weiland S. Family care giving at home, *Home Health Care Nurse* 2002;**20**(2): 113–9.
8   Bjornsdottir K. From the state to the family: reconfiguring the responsibility on long term nursing care at home. *Nurs Inquiry* 2002;**9**:3–11.
9   Edwards B. Quality of life instruments for caregivers of patients with cancer: A review of their psychometric properties. *Cancer Nurs* 2002;**25**:342–9.

10 Cousineau N, McDowell I, Hotz S, Hebert Pl. Measuring chronic patients' feelings of being a burden to their caregivers: Development and preliminary validation of a scale. *Med Care* 2003;**41**:110–18.
11 Krause N, Borawski-Clark E. Clarifying the functions of social support. *Res Ageing* 1994;**16**:251–79.
12 Glasgow Joint Carers Strategy 2002–2005. www.Glasgow.gov.uk/html/council/dept/social/jycr.pdf (accessed 19 November 2003).

Index

Page numbers in **bold** text refer to figures in the text; those in *italics* refer to tables or boxes